Foreword

When the authors asked me to write the foreword for this book, I did feel privileged and honored. When one looks at the scope and content of this book, you could easily deduce that the combination of the knowledge and experience of these two authors would do great justice to the book and subjects covered.

The book tries to make up for several aspects of health care which were not addressed when the curriculum was formed and subsequently amended from time to time. This includes new responsibilities for dental surgeons in view of the enormous strides in the specialty in the last few decades. Some of these include responsibilities like hospital dentistry, treatment of medically compromised patients with multiple drug histories, and even the possibility of grave morbidity or mortality one may encounter.

The issues pertaining to emergencies, disability and death and its consequences is something most medical professionals let alone dental surgeons are ill qualified to do. The declaration of death and cause of death has been the subject of much a debate.

It is hoped that with better documentation and paperwork pertaining to accidents, injuries, wound/death certification and autopsies will enable seamless legal proceedings in cases of unnatural or unexpected clinic/ hospital death. This will also prevent emotional outbursts by the public resulting in violence against health professionals.

"Physician, heal thyself" is a commonly used phrase. Never has a truer word been said. We have the absolute moral and ethical duty to protect our patients and prevent any untoward consequences to them. We are the defenders of the faith they repose in us. Complications happen. Their incidence can certainly be reduced but tragically never be prevented. The book provides scope for training and auditing outcomes to prevent recurrence or mitigate complications

Autopsy and Forensics have been given a niche space within the contents. That really sums up the completeness and conciseness of what the authors have attempted. The findings on an autopsy table will be as useful to us as the information obtained from treating thousands of 'live" patients. Autopsies and forensics are not routinely taught within dental curricula and perhaps only cursorily covered at medical schools and colleges. Forensic odontology has acquired great importance as the protection of the pulp by the density of the teeth allows the extraction of DNA for identification and criminal investigation. This is surely possible as an addition in subsequent editions to prove wrong the idiom "dead men tell no tales".

I hope this book will be a brilliant addition to the repertoire of literature available on the subject of critical medical care, documentation, and forensics for dental surgeons.

Kishore Nayak
MDS FDSRCS (Eng) FFFRCS (Irel.) FDSRCPS (Glas)
Past President Association of Oral and Maxillofacial Surgeons of India
Past President International Association of Oral and Maxillofacial Surgeons
Honorary Fellow American Association of Oral and Maxillofacial Surgeons
Honorary Fellow Australia New Zealand Association of Oral and Maxillofacial Surgeons
Honorary Fellow South African Association of Oral and Maxillofacial Surgeons
Honorary Fellow of the International Board of Certification of Specialists in
Oral and Maxillofacial Surgery
Honorary Fellow of the Indian Board of Oral and Maxillofacial Surgery.

Manual of Procedures for Emergencies, Morbidity and Mortality in Dental Outpatient and Hospital Practice

Dr Manikandhan R

MDS FDSRCS FFDRCS MNAMS

Dr George Paul

MDS DNB LLB Dip. MLE

Illustrations by

Dr J Balaji

MDS MBA

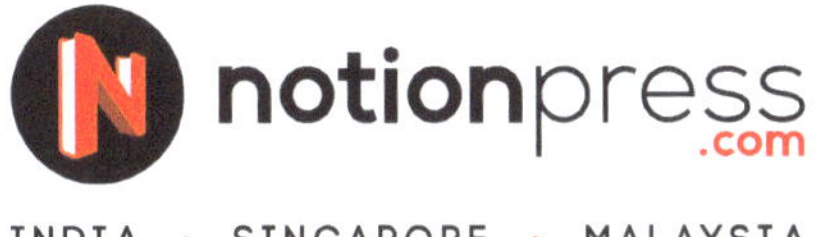

Preface

This book is slightly different from standard textbooks or subject guides in that it covers a wide range of subjects. The book is designed to fill up the gaps in the dental curriculum that were not hitherto addressed. Rapid advances in Dental Surgery, and the ambit of their work has made it necessary that they are better equipped to handle complex outcomes in the best interest of patient safety.

This is particularly so in the surgical specialities like Oral and Maxillofacial Surgery which is a recognised speciality of dentistry involved in trauma, cancer, TMJ surgeries and cosmetic basal bone procedures. Some of them can be done exclusively only by these surgeons. Dental surgeons too are increasingly using sedation and anaesthetics to perform minor surgery like implants and dento-alveolar procedures.

This book will hopefully encourage the national dental commission to introduce subjects such as training in emergency medicine and dealing with life-saving procedures. In the unfortunate event of morbidity or mortality Dental Surgeons must necessarily possess knowledge in recognizing these situations, instituting emergency procedures and declaring/ certifying cause of death.

The book has several chapters dealing with relevant topics and offers information like general forensic medicine and statutory requirements in case of unnatural or natural death reporting.

We hope the book will serve as a hand book for clinicians and a textbook for undergraduate and post graduate students.

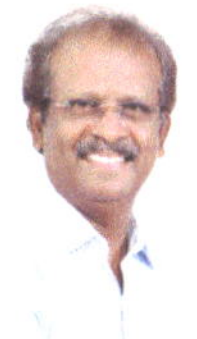

Dr. Manikandhan R
MDS FDSRCS FFDRCS MNAMS

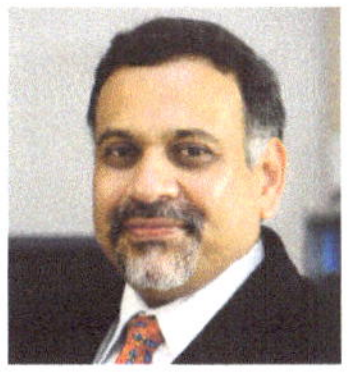

Dr. George Paul
MDS DNB LLB Dip. MLE

Acknowledgements

Writing a unique book was harder than I thought, as it needed everything new and to be created from scratch. It took almost a couple of years of hard work to complete this write-up as I spoke to colleagues and well-wishers about the idea of the book. I wish to thank the first persons who gave momentum to this book: my two young surgeons at that time, Dr. Raj and Dr. Kumaran, who started pouring me with essential articles and some ideas.

My heartfelt sincere thanks go to Prof. Dr. George Paul, a co-author of this book, since this book also has major components of law and ethics, and I couldn't think of a better person other than him. He gave lots of ideas on what to include and exclude to make it absolutely necessary for the practitioners to use it as a reference manual.

I also wish to thank Prof. Dr. J. Balaji who made some beautiful illustrations for every chapter with a little wit in them to make the book more attractive. It was completely an honorary work by him as a commitment to this book.

My heartfelt thanks go out to Dr. Sailesh Kumar, who was my cleft fellow and took exceptional pain and time to create new diagrams and photographs, which are more self-explanatory.

Thanks to Dr. Kavitha Bottu, HOD of the Dept. of Oral Pathology, Dr. Ramya Sekar, Dr. Sathya Priya, and Dr. Samuel Thomas faculties, who contributed a beautiful chapter on forensic odontology.

Dr. Elavenil, who is a very eminent scholar and surgeon, was instrumental in content editing, grammar checks, and sentence rephrasing. I wish to thank her for the immense effort and input for the final finish of the book. Thanks to Dr. Ritvi Bagadia and Dr. Anandhi Visweswaran, my surgical fellows and clinical associates, for their contributions in proof reading and editing.

I also thank Dr. Saravanan from Coimbatore for contributing a part of a chapter on emergencies and Dr. Kiran from Salem for contributing wonderful hand-drawn diagrams for one of the chapters.

I want to thank Dr. Marieas publications and Research International PVT LTD for their great contributions in doing some referencing and content correction.

Thanks to my department faculty and trainees for their constant support and encouragement for the entire 3 years. I will be failing in my duty if I fail to mention the immense support given by our interim chancellor, pro-chancellor, vice chancellor, pro-vice chancellor, and dean of research at MAHER University, Chennai. I extend my sincere thanks to Central Library MAHER University for extending their support in providing us with plagiarism checking by Turnitin software.

Heartfelt thanks to Dr. Suvy Manuel Maxillofacial surgeon and, a scientific writing scholar, for adding precision to the textbook with his wonderful editing and proof reading.

Special thanks to all my teachers from India and abroad, and specifically my beloved teacher and mentor, Prof. Dr. Kishore Nayak, who consented and wrote a wonderful foreword for this book.

Lastly, I wish to thank my wife, Dr. Nirupa, and daughter, Dr. Nikita, for their sustained support in ways that I never knew that I needed. I wish to thank my dear daughter, Dr. Nikita, an ophthalmologist, and Dr. Keerthi, a trainee OMFS, for adding the final colors for the front cover picture and adding input into ophthalmology diagrams.

My heartfelt thanks to everyone who ever said anything positive to me or taught me something. Finally, I want to thank the Almighty, because without God, I wouldn't be able to do any of this work.

We wish to thank generously the effort taken by the Notion press team from the start of this work in accepting, language copyediting, technical editing, typeset proof and meeting the target time in every aspect of publishing this book.

Authors

Main Authors:

1. Dr. Manikandhan Ramanathan
MDS FDSRCS FFDRCS MNAMS
Senior Professor
Dept of Oral and Maxillofacial Surgery

Director
Meenakshi Institute of Facial Aesthetics and
Craniofacial Excellence (MIFACE)
Meenakshi Dental College and Hospital
MAHER University
Chennai

Dean
International relations
MAHER University
K K Nagar
Chennai

2. Dr. George Paul
MDS DNB LLB Dip. MLE
Senior consultant Oral and Maxillofacial
Surgeon,
Dr. Paulose Memorial Dental Clinic, Salem.
Chairman, Advisory Committee, Sharon
Palliative Centre, Salem
Adjunct Professor, DY Patil Dental College
and Hospital, Pune
Chairman, Institutional Review Board, Salem
Polyclinic, Salem

Formerly:
Professor, Department of Oral and
Maxillofacial Surgery, VMS Dental college,
Salem
Past Hon. Adjunct Professor, Dr. MGR
Medical University (2011-2016)
Member, Faculty of Dentistry, Kerala
University of Health Sciences (2018-2021)
Past President AOMSI (2009-2010)
Past Hon. Secretary AOMSI (2003- 2006)

Contributors

Dr. B Kavitha MDS
Professor and HOD
Dept. of Oral and Maxillofacial Pathology
Meenakshi Ammal dental college and
hospital
Chennai.

Dr. J Balaji MDS MBA
Professor
Dept. of Oral and Maxillofacial surgery
Tamilnadu Government Dental College and
Hospital
Chennai

Dr. A I Raj MDS
Associate Professor
Dept. of Oral and Maxillofacial Surgery
Meenakshi Ammal Dental College and
Hospital
MAHER University
Chennai

Dr. Sailesh Kumar MDS FCLPCS
Assistant Professor
Dept. of OMFS
Indira Gandhi Institute of Dental Sciences
Sri Balaji Vidyapeeth
Puducherry

Prof. Dr. Elavenil MDS MBA
FDSRCPS(Glasgow)
Dept. of Oral and Maxillofacial Surgery
SRM dental college
SRM university
Ramapuram
Chennai

Dr. Anandhi Visweswaran MDS
Research Associate and Cleft Fellow
Meenakshi Institute of Facial Aesthetics and
Craniofacial Excellence,
MAHER university
Chennai

Dr. Ramya Sekar MDS
Assistant Professor
Dept of Oral and Maxillofacial Pathology
Meenakshi Ammal Dental College and
Hospital
Chennai

Dr. Samuel Thomas MDS
Assistant Professor
Dept. Of Oral and Maxillofacial Pathology
Shree bankee Bihari Dental College
Ghaziabad
Uttar Pradesh

Dr. Sathya Priya MDS
Assistant Professor
Dept. of Oral and Maxillofacial Pathology
Meenakshi Ammal Dental College and
Hospital
Chennai

Dr. Ritvi MDS FCLPCS
Assistant professor
Sri Ramachandra Dental college and Hospital
Sri Ramachandra University
Porur
Chennai

Dr. Mariea Francis MDS PhD
Oral and Maxillofacial Surgeon
Assistant professor
KVG Dental College and Hospital
Sullia
Karnataka

Dr. Suvy Manuel MDS, DNB, MNAMS,
MFDS RCS Eng, MOS RCSEd,
FDS RCS Ed
Oral and maxillofacial surgeon.
The Oral Surgery office, Trivandrum

Dr. M Kumaran MDS
Oral and Maxillofacial Surgeon
Director
Floss and Gloss Dental Care
Chennai

Glossary

Definition of Legal and Technical Terms

Act – Any law passed by the legislature and assented to by the President of India or Governor of State

Bill – A Bill is a draft of law moved or to be moved before parliament or legislature. A Bill when passed becomes an Act.

Law – The system of rules which a particular country or community recognizes as regulating the actions of its members and which it may enforce by the imposition of penalties.

Legality – The quality or state of being in accordance with the law.

Justice – Justice is the legal or philosophical theory by which fairness is administered.

Court – A body of people presided over by a judge, judges, or magistrate, and acting as a tribunal in civil and criminal cases.

Municipality – A town or district that has local government.

VAO – Village Administrative Officer (India) Tehsildar (in India) A collector for, or official of, the revenue department.

Death – The action or fact of dying or being killed; the end of the life of a person or organism.

Disability – A disadvantage or handicap, especially one imposed or recognized by the law

Deformity – The state of being deformed or misshapen

RBD – Registrar of Births and Death

RBD Act 1969 – An Act to provide for the regulation of registration of births and deaths and for matters connected therewith.

Medical Negligence – An act or omission (failure to act) by a medical professional that deviates from the accepted medical standard of care.

Civil and Criminal Liability – Potential responsibility for payment of damages or other court-enforcement in a lawsuit, as distinguished from criminal liability, which means open to punishment for a crime.

Statutory Liability – is a legal term indicating the liability of a party who may be held responsible for any action or omission due to a related law that is not open to interpretation.

Indian Penal Code 1860	–	The Indian Penal Code (IPC) is the main criminal code of India. It is a comprehensive code intended to cover all substantive aspects of criminal law.
Consumer Protection Act 1986	–	A state or federal law designed to protect consumers against improperly described, damaged, faulty, and dangerous goods and services as well as unfair trade and credit practices.
Evidence Act (India)	–	The Indian Evidence Act, originally passed in India by the Imperial Legislative Council in 1872, during the British Raj, contains a set of rules and allied issues governing the admissibility of evidence in the Indian courts of law.
Forensic Medicine	–	The branch of medicine dealing with the application of medical knowledge to establish facts in civil or criminal legal cases, such as an investigation into the cause and time of a suspicious death.
Forensic Odontology	–	A branch of forensic medicine dealing with teeth and marks left by teeth (as in identifying criminal suspects or the remains of a dead person)
MCCD	–	Medical Certification for Cause of Death
Death Certificate	–	A Death Certificate is a document issued by the Government to the nearest relatives of the deceased, stating the date, fact, and cause of death. It is essential to register death to prove the time and date of death, to establish the fact of death for relieving the individual from social, legal, and official obligations, to enable settlement of property inheritance, and to authorise the family to collect insurance and other benefits.
Disability Certificate	–	The Disability Certificate is not just a document for a person with a disability but a proof of his/her disability and an important tool for availing the benefits / facilities / rights that they are entitled to, from the Central as well as State Government under various appropriate enabling legislations.
FIR	–	A First Information Report (FIR) is a written document prepared by police organizations in countries like India when they receive information about the commission of a cognisable offense
CSR	–	For a non-cognizable offense, a Community Service Register is created & registered in the Police station
CGHS	–	Central Government Health Scheme
WHO	–	World Health Organization
AIIMS	–	All India Institute of Medical Sciences

Contents

Introduction - Why This Book?

Every healthcare system in the world has a special position for dentistry. In contemporary medicine, it is a distinct field of study. The treatment of dental and oral disorders only in the recent past became a part of an integrative system that included holistic health care, though, when one considers that contemporary medical systems are only a little more than a century old.

In the evolution of modern medicine, the specialization of dentistry as an independent profession is an accident and an aberration. The initial dentists were actually physicians with a specialty in managing dental and oral problems.

Early in the twentieth century, dental institutions and curricula were created as distinct from medical colleges, and the division of the two fields of study spread to other nations. We must evaluate dentistry's growth from this perspective, especially given that stomatology, which includes dentistry, is the only anatomically separate entity that does not develop into a post-medical speciality like ophthalmology, otorhinolaryngology, or gastroenterology.

Dentistry started out more as an art, which involved the restoration and replacement of teeth and general care of the mouth. The only surgical aspect was the extraction of teeth, which evolved from a rather gruesome proposition in the pre-local anaesthesia era to a more scientific procedure with the advent of modern anaesthetics and analgesics. However, rapid advances in oral surgery and invasive dental surgery made it necessary for dentists to reintegrate into their former medical backgrounds.

In order to better prepare the dental graduate to comprehend and perform the speciality as a part of contemporary health care, significant modifications to the dental school's curriculum were made by adding a number of fundamental medical and clinical disciplines.[1] Over the next few decades, several critical aspects of surgery in the oral and peri-oral regions, such as maxillofacial trauma and pathologies involving the oral cavity, fell into the ambit of the dental surgeon, who was strategically better equipped to treat conditions.

The two world wars and subsequent conflicts, in which dental and oral surgeons were discovered to be helpful in the treatment of face bone fractures, largely supplied encouragement. Thus, Temporomandibular joint (TMJ) procedures, surgical repairs of dentofacial abnormalities, and aesthetic surgery of the face are only a few of the surgical specialties that now fall under the umbrella of oral and maxillofacial surgery.[2,3]

To better handle surgical management and treatment in a complex area of the body where one needs a thorough grasp of both medical and surgical principles and dental ideas, this dictated the necessity of dual qualifications (medical and dental) in numerous nations, including Europe.[4] Oral and maxillofacial surgery is still a surgical speciality of dentistry in various countries, including the USA, India, and other Asian nations. It needs to be kept in mind that oral and maxillofacial surgeons (OMFS) with dental training continue to provide care for 90% of the world's population. The USA, Canada, Latin America, the Caribbean, the majority of African nations, China, Central Asia, South Asia, Middle East Asia, South West Asia, Japan, and Far East Asia are among those that fall under this category.

Dentistry, in general, became a cutting-edge medical specialty with advances in conscious sedation, extensive periodontal surgery, the management of patients with medical co-morbidities, and the rehabilitation of disabilities and deformities of the gnathological system (jaws).

In the early years of dentistry in India, aggressive and invasive procedures with multiple drugs were not conceived as part of routine dentistry. With a significant change in the profile of work done by dental/oral and maxillofacial surgeons, patient safety and comprehensive medical knowledge became imperative for all practitioners, particularly those doing surgery and dental procedures under general anaesthesia.

The curriculum has been suitably modified to include patient safety, and training has prepared dentists to tackle life-threatening conditions. However, the Dentist Act of 1948 did not anticipate death and serious morbidity as a possible sequel to dental procedures, however rare they may be. The current dental curriculum is preparing dentists to understand grievous or fatal outcomes

and is training them in basic and advanced life support. It has therefore become necessary to anticipate the unlikely possibility of morbidity, disability, or death while undergoing treatment for dental and oral conditions.[5]

This book also deals with several gaps in the training of dental surgeons as full-fledged health professionals with the autonomy to prescribe, admit, request investigations, and order transfusions, in addition to doing surgery in the mouth and facial bones amongst other things. The dental and oral surgeon is expected to recognize, intervene, and perform emergency life-saving measures and deal with outcomes including death and forensic procedures.

The Dental Council of India Code of Ethics regulation of 2014 (under 10.5), has recognized the need for dentists to be prepared to recognize death and take steps in such events after the approval from central government. The code has now entrusted the dentist with the responsibility of declaring death and issuing certificate to that effect, if the patient was in the care of a dental or oral and maxillofacial surgeon.

As the statutes were silent on this issue until recently, the authors have outlined procedures that need to be addressed in this unlikely event and the procedures required by law to declare and report the cause of death to the agencies responsible.

The authors have included chapters dealing with emergencies, their management, reporting and managing injuries, their quantification, the pathophysiology of death and clinical signs for identification of death, declaring death, issuing medical certification for the cause of death (MCCD), whenever known and deemed necessary, and reporting such events to the statutory body or investigating agencies.

References:

1. BDS course regulations by Dental council of India **http://www.dciindia. org.in/Rule_Regulation/Revised_BDS_ Course_Regulation_2007.pdf**
2. Field MJ, Editor. Dental education at the crossroads: challenges and change (1995)
3. Rahul Tiwari et al. History of Oral and Maxillofacial Surgery – A Review. IOSR Journal of Dental and Medical Sciences (IOSR-JDMS). Volume 16, Issue 3 Ver. VIII (March. 2017), PP 99-102
4. Martin-Granizo R. Double degree in oral and maxillofacial surgery—is it necessary? International Journal of Oral and Maxillofacial Surgery. 2017 Mar 1; 46:34.
5. Revised Dentists (Code of Ethics) Regulations – 2014, Part II, Section 3, Sub-sec (1) of the Gazette of India

Common Medical Emergencies in Dental Office

2.1 Introduction

Life-threatening emergencies tend to happen in a dental set-up. When it does, it is assumed that the dentist and his or her team will be able to manage a potentially fatal condition until the patient is transferred to a medical institution using the fundamental skills. It is a dentist's responsibility to handle these events and, hence be trained and equipped to handle such emergency management procedures.[1] This chapter seeks to give a general overview of dental crises and how to handle them. (Figure 2.1 a)

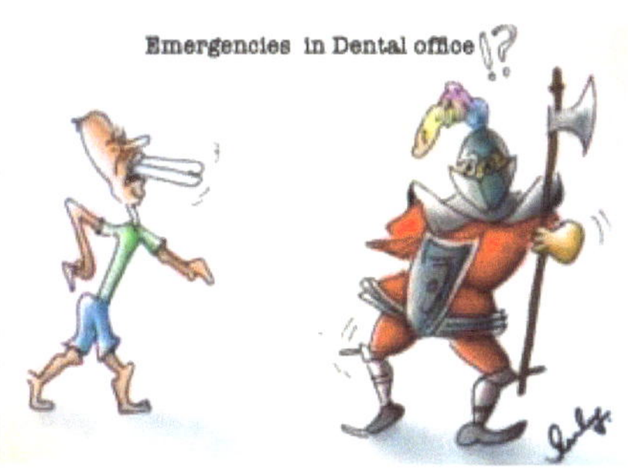

Figure 2.1 a: Emergencies in a dental office

The following section provides details on how some typical medical situations are handled in dentistry offices.

2.2 Common Medical Emergencies

2.2.1 Vasovagal Syncope

Syncope is defined as a sudden and transient loss of consciousness with spontaneous recovery. It is an autonomic reaction that causes broad blood vessel dilation in the splanchnic and skeletal arteries as well as bradycardia, which reduces brain perfusion.

Signs and symptoms of vasovagal syncope: This includes pallor, nausea, sweating, blurred vision, and unconsciousness.

Management:
The patient is made to lie in a flat position with raised legs. Oxygen is administered. The patient is maintained in a supine position and re-assured until the heart rate and blood pressure return to normal.[1] In situations where syncope is prolonged or accompanied by seizures or the patient has a history of any other medical complications, the patient must be immediately transferred to a hospital setup, for any further management.

2.2.2 Angina Pectoris

Angina pectoris is characterized by central or left-sided chest pain. It is a medical disorder characterized by frequent episodes of discomfort and pain brought on by an imbalance between the oxygen delivery and requirements of the myocardium. Some of the causes of angina that result in altered myocardial metabolism and pain are constriction by spasm, narrowing by coronary sclerosis, or occlusion by a thrombus or inadequate coronary blood supply. The pain caused by angina pectoris may be acutely severe and excruciating; it is usually felt as generalized pressure over the chest or under the sternum. In some cases, the pain may even be felt in the teeth, lower jaw, clavicle, and shoulders, radiating down the left or both arms. Angina attacks are usually of short duration, lasting less than 2–3 minutes, and are triggered by exertion, excessive eating, or some form of emotional excitement. Severe dental anxiety and acute pain during dental procedures can also induce coronary spasms.

Management:
Acute anginal attacks in dental chair may be precipitated due to acute pain/ stress and or unstable angina which the patient may be already having.

- reassurance and loosening of tight garments
- immediate cessation of all dental procedures
- position patient comfortably and oxygen can be administered immediately
- sublingual nitroglycerine tablet or spray (up to 3 doses)
- expected time for improvement is 3 minutes

Wait for the pain to get relieved, if not seek medical help immediately with monitors on. The primary objective in these emergencies is to reduce the chance of developing myocardial infarction or death rather than negate with continuation of treatment.

2.2.3 Myocardial Infarction-MI

Although rare in dental chair, patient may develop left sided chest pain with or without radiation to left arm. Constrictive left sided chest pain not subsided by nitroglycerine in emergency is a good indicator of MI. Patient may vomit, sweat and lose consciousness with lose of pulse and breathing.

Management:
- cessation of all dental treatments
- position patient in upright or semi reclined position
- encourage patient to chew Aspirin 375mg immediately
- administer oxygen 5L/minute with monitoring of vital signs
- If patient becomes unresponsive with no breathing and pulse, consider diagnosis of cardiac arrest
- Consider CPCR and seek medical help with hospital transfer in monitor

2.2.4 Epileptic Fit

Tonic-clonic seizure in dental chair may be precipitated by various factors of stress, hypoxia and missing medication if taking regularly.

Major seizure:
In addition to jerking motions of the head, arms, and legs, there is an abrupt

spasm of muscular stiffness (tonic phase). In addition to having loud or spasmodic breathing, salivation, and incontinence, the person may also go unconscious. The prodromal phase, which is not a seizure but rather a change in mood or behavior, is included in this. There might be an aura right before a fit. This is a characteristic of a seizure and has been described as a "strange feeling in the gut," an unusual scent, or flashing lights.

Management:
The patient is moved away from dangerous objects and made to lie flat. Then the patient is turned into the recovery position. Recovery is checked every 5 minutes. If recovery is good, the patient is reassured and discharged with a family member. If not, status epilepticus must be considered. Emergency Medical Service (EMS) is alerted, and high-flow O_2 is administered. Midazolam is administered buccally or intranasally: 10mg for adults and children >10 years; 7.5mg for children between 5 and 10 years; or Diazepam 10mg IV over two minutes (2.5mg over 30 seconds).

mental function, mood fluctuations, reduced spontaneity, hunger, and nausea.

- sweating, tachycardia, piloerection, nervousness, strange behavioural patterns, poor judgment are signs of "severe stage"
- the "more severe stage" is marked by coma, hypotension, hypothermia, seizures, and unconsciousness.

Management:
For a conscious patient, oral glucose is administered. Upon recovery, the patient is discharged. If unsuccessful, EMS (Emergency Medical Services under National Rural Health Mission) is activated. 25% dextrose is administered by IV as fast as possible, or Glucagon 1mg is given subcutaneously or intramuscularly. The patient is monitored and discharged upon recovery. For an unconscious patient, the following basic steps are followed: airway, breathing, circulation, and definitive management. IV 50% dextrose solution/1 mg glucagon is administered by parenteral route. [3]

2.2.5 Hypoglycemia

Hypoglycemia is a condition when the blood glucose level falls below the threshold of 40 mg/dL for children and 50 mg/dL for adults. It is possible for people without diabetes to develop this disease.

Symptoms and signs of hypoglycemia:
The description of each stage of hypoglycemia is provided below.
- a modest response known as the "early stage" is characterized by diminished

2.2.6 Asthma

The most prevalent chronic, non-transmittable respiratory condition impacting people of all ages and racial origins is asthma. With the possibility of an abrupt exacerbation, asthma is a diverse chronic inflammatory disorder of the lungs that is marked by airway constriction and hypersecretion. Allergies, infections, anxiety, etc. can cause this.

Clinical signs and symptoms of acute asthma exacerbations:
These include expiratory wheezing, shortness of breath, coughing, and chest tightness. Less commonly, it causes fatigue, dizziness, and lightheadedness. Life-threatening signs and symptoms include severe dyspnea, a slow respiratory rate, cyanosis, drowsiness, confusion, and bradycardia.

Management:
The patient is placed upright in a comfortable position. Any ongoing surgical procedure is paused and the oral cavity should be kept free of any instruments / dental materials (restorative materials, cotton etc). Watch for chest rise and pay attention to breath sounds in awake individuals, to ensure the patency of airway. EMS is activated. Two deep inhalations of fast-acting bronchodilators (albuterol and salbutamol) are dispensed. In the case of an unresponsive patient, IM injection of adrenaline (0.1 ml per 10 kg body weight of adrenaline 1mg/ml) is administered along with oxygen at a flow rate of 5 to 6 L/min. In case of a delay in shifting to a hospital, Inj Hydrocortisone sodium succinate 100mg IV is administered.

2.2.7 Choking

Foreign body obstruction of the airway, or FBAO, is a frequent and sometimes fatal complication in dentistry. The foreign body frequently encountered are dentures, endodontic files / tooth etc. Rescue missions are typically carried out while the choking sufferer is still alert and aware.

Signs and symptoms:
The universal choking signal includes difficult, paradoxical breathing that lacks voice or air movement and raises blood pressure, heart rate, and other symptoms, including losing consciousness.

Management:
The patient is placed in a lateral decubitus position and encouraged to cough. Other manual, non-invasive procedures include manual thrust, which is a series of thrusts to the upper abdomen (Heimlich maneuver or abdominal thrust). If the patient becomes unconscious, the ABCDE approach is followed.

2.2.8 Anaphylaxis

Anaphylaxis is a life-threatening medical emergency. The presentation can range from severe airway blockage, convulsions to death in a matter of minutes if left undiagnosed. The other most frequent findings include urticaria and angioedema (87%), wheezing or shortness of breath (59%), and signs of hypotension (33%)[5].

Anaphylaxis must be diagnosed when two or more of the signs and symptoms listed below manifest suddenly (within minutes to hours): skin-mucosal involvement, difficulty breathing, hypotension and related symptoms, and prolonged gastrointestinal problems. It's also critical to be mindful of the possibility of biphasic responses which denotes recurrence of symptoms after a short duration of normalcy. Less than 1% to 20% of anaphylaxis cases are accompanied by biphasic responses[4] which mandates 24 hours monitoring.

Management:
Evaluation of the airway, breathing, circulation, and awareness are required. Anaphylaxis symptoms and indicators are examined in the digestive and cutaneous systems. Any ongoing procedures are stopped, the patient's airway is cleansed of debris, and any possible triggers are taken away. If the patient is having trouble breathing, they are placed supine or sitting up with their legs raised. Sustain oxygen flow at 5 to 6 L/min, epinephrine 0.3 to 0.5 mg/1:1000 is injected intramuscularly or subcutaneously, 25–50 mg of Diphenhydramine, and 100 mg of Hydrocortisone sodium succinate are administered IM/ IV as required every 5–10 minutes. At least 6–8 L/min of additional oxygen is provided via a facemask in the interim. Vital signs are continuously monitored, and if breathing stops, basic life support is started. If symptoms continue, IM adrenaline is re-administered every 5 minutes. Adrenaline 1:1000 (1mg/ml) is injected intramuscularly at a dose of 0.5 ml for patients >16 years, 0.15 ml for children under 6 years, 0.3 ml for children between 6 - 12 years, 0.5 ml for patients between 12-16 years.[5,6]

2.2.9 Hyperventilation

Hyperventilation is "an increased exchange of air due to deepened respiration, an increased rate of respiration, or both."

Signs and symptoms:
Breathing deeply and quickly, tingling in the fingers or lips, tetanic spasms in the periphery, and lightheadedness. Relative cerebral hypoxia can cause unconsciousness to set in.

Management:
The patient is placed, comforted, and the airway is kept open. Simple breathing exercises or breathing into a paper bag can also be helpful since they increase the amount of carbon dioxide that is inspired. If the patient becomes unconscious, the airway is kept open, and they are placed in the recovery position until they become cognizant again.[7]

2.2.10 Adrenal Crisis

An endocrine condition known as adrenal insufficiency (AI) is defined by the adrenal cortex's insufficient synthesis of adrenal androgens, mineralocorticoids, and glucocorticoids. It is of two types: primary and secondary adrenal insufficiency. It frequently results from the gradual destruction of the adrenal cortex, which is typically idiopathic in nature (most frequently, autoimmune). However, it can also be brought on by hemorrhage, sepsis, infectious illnesses (like tuberculosis, human immunodeficiency virus, cytomegalovirus, and fungal infection), malignancy, adrenalectomy, amyloidosis, the use of certain drugs, or congenital disorders. For people who need surgical dental care, the circumstances are less clear; therefore, it makes sense to make sure they are covered until further information is made accessible.

In general, risk reduction in high-risk patients can be accomplished by planning their scheduled procedures in the morning when endogenous cortisol levels are higher, making sure they have taken their usual steroid dose prior to the procedure, and if required, offering adequate analgesia and anxiety medications.

Signs and symptoms:
Confusion, perspiration, nausea, diarrhoea, hypotension, loss of consciousness, convulsions, and finally circulatory collapse are some of these symptoms.

Management:
The O_2 flow is increased. Emergency services are notified, and the patient is in a supine posture. Provide 100 mg hydrocortisone IV/IM followed by 200 mg over the next 24 hours given IM/IV (50 mg every 6 hours) or as a continuous infusion. The patient undergoes hospitalization if necessary.

2.3 Conclusion

Any clinician who works in a dental clinic may find medical crisis scary, but with the right measures and the required training, these circumstances tend to be less worrisome. Despite the rarity of serious medical issues during dental treatments, dentist must be prepared to address them. The dentist is primarily responsible for managing an emergency situation effectively at the dental office. Medical crises should be handled at the office by all healthcare professionals, who should be trained to do so.

References

1. Malamed FS. Medical emergencies in the dental office, ed 6, St. Louis, Mosby. 2007
2. Lowenstein DH, Bleck T, Macdonald RL. It's time to revise the definition of status epilepticus.. 1999
3. Bavitz JB. Emergency management of hypoglycemia and hyperglycemia. Dent Clin North Am. 1995;39(3):587-94.
4. Tole JW, Lieberman P. Biphasic anaphylaxis: review of incidence, clinical predictors, and observation recommendations. Immunology and allergy clinics of North America. 2007 May 1;27(2):309-26.
5. Webb L, Greene E, Lieberman PL. Anaphylaxis: a review of 593 cases. Journal of Allergy and Clinical Immunology. 2004 Feb 1;113(2): S240.
6. Freeman TM. Anaphylaxis: diagnosis and treatment. Prim Care 1998; 25:809–81
7. Lazarus, H., and Kostan, J. Psychogenic hyperventilation and death anxiety. Psychosomatic 10:14-22,1969

Guidelines for Training of Dental Specialists in Basic Resuscitation Course and Emergency Management

3.1 Introduction

We have always been told, as dental surgeons, that there is an emergency lurking behind every compromised or even regular patient. Remember, "an emergency will never announce itself. When it happens, it might be too late to think of possibilities. Management of emergencies is based on continuous training and anticipation."

Dental surgery training has large lacunae regarding the recognition and management of medical emergencies in clinical practice. As already discussed, dental training is slowly filling up these inadequacies by re-formatting the curriculum to provide better knowledge and improve the safety of the patient in a clinical situation. Today, we see a need for training in recognition of morbid situations, emergency management, certification of outcomes, etc., when dealing with situations that may arise in a medical outpatient or inpatient facility. A new generation of older patients living with many co-morbid conditions has made the Dental Council review its syllabus, curriculum, and certifying responsibilities. This includes the introduction of new subjects and modified syllabus to meet these challenges. This chapter serves to familiarize the dental surgeon with subjects such as emergency medicine, surgery, and forensic pathology.

3.1.1 So Where Do We Start to Be Competent?

In our opinion, every dental specialist must have a comprehensive basic medical curriculum commensurate with the demands of today's medical practice. The basic syllabus and curriculum must be upgraded for the first- and second-year students to understand the clinical scenarios that they can expect to encounter in the later years. More importantly, it should form the basis for understanding the key aspects of medical management for the dental patient, particularly in an emergency.

The curriculum should also include topics that have so far been excluded due to the false notion that they are irrelevant. This includes emergency medicine in the form of mandatory training in basic and advanced CPR and Advanced Cardiac Life Support (ACLS), with the necessity to periodically upgrade even after qualification. It is also mandatory to reinforce the curriculum to include general forensic pathology in addition to the current narrow spectrum of forensic odontology.

It is needless to say those specialties in hospital dentistry, such as oral and maxillofacial surgery or oral medicine and pedodontics, must have postgraduate programs that impart the necessary skills to deal with extremely sick or medically vulnerable patients.

Medical situations that might result in significant morbidity and death could affect any dental practitioner or dental care professional. We are aware that medical emergencies occur more than what is reported because we do not report them in India as is done in western countries, where it is mandatory and audited regularly.

Some of the conditions that may produce intra-operative or post-operative mortality include myocardial infarction, choking, severe asthma, epileptic attacks, high sedation, and anaphylaxis. Of course, general anaesthesia-related complications are a large spectrum of conditions that will have serious implications for oral and maxillofacial surgeons and Pedodontists.

Every dental practice in India ought to provide staff training on how to handle such circumstances. To develop cooperation, dental teams should take part in frequent training that replicates crises. It will also be ideal if the Dental Council of India (DCI) convenes a working party and frames guidelines for training dentists to gain competency for safeguarding the lives of patients.

3.2 'ABCDE' approach

All working staff in the dental clinic should be alerted once the patient is sick' and likely to have a morbidity or collapse. Constant vigilance should be exercised at all times to detect any medical emergency by recognizing an abnormal breathing pattern, an abnormal patient colour (pale or bluish), an abnormal pulse rate, etc. This enables the right assistance to be called, such as an ambulance/EMS, before any patient passes out.

The 'ABCDE' principles-based systematic approach to treating critically ill patients is promoted. Proper documentation and knowledge of the patient's medical history should also make it possible to identify those who are "at risk" for specific medical emergencies and refer them appropriately, which may call for delaying the recommended treatment or recommending that it be received in a hospital.

3.3 General Principles

3.3.1 Patient Collapses in the Dental Chair

1. The ABCDE strategy (airway, breathing, circulation, disability, and exposure) is used to evaluate and treat the patient.
2. Before going on to the next stage of the examination, life-threatening

issues are handled when they are observed first.

3. If there is additional worsening, re-evaluation is conducted continuously, beginning with the airway.

4. Any treatment's results are evaluated.

5. The need for extra help must be recognized and help must be sought early. (Ambulance 108 for emergencics)

6. The dental team as a whole must be utilized.to accomplish many tasks at once, such as gathering equipment and medications for emergencies.

7. The team must be properly structured and communicative.

8. The goals of initial care are to maintain the patient's life, bring about some clinical improvement, and create time for follow-up care while awaiting assistance.

9. It should be kept in mind that therapy may take a few minutes to take effect.

10. The ABCDE method may be applied by anybody, regardless of their background or expertise in clinical evaluation or therapy.

3.3.2 Possible Reasons for Mortality in Dentistry

1. Heavy sedation in a dental clinic with inadequate expertise and infrastructure to manage emergency.

2. Sedation and local anaesthesia

3. Pre-existing severe cardiovascular pathology

4. Wrong drug injection during GA or during emergencies

5. Severe bleeding from underlying disorders after tooth extractions

6. Airway obstruction from aspiration, pneumonia, or foreign body aspiration

7. Infective endocarditis secondary to dental invasive procedures.

8. Severe septicemia patients admitted as inpatients due to dental causes

9. Hyperthyroid crisis and overdose/toxicity secondary to local anaesthesia injection with adrenaline

10. Debilitating and handicapped patients treated in dental chairs` with sedation with underlying medical co-morbidities.

11. Unexpected cardiac arrest with no obvious reason

3.4 Training in CPCR

In the European and American continents, almost all dentists and healthcare professionals undergo compulsory Cardio Pulmonary Cerebral Resuscitation (CPCR) training during their study period as well as during clinical practice, at least once every 2 years. It is important to keep up the knowledge in an ever-changing scenario in the medical field regarding the management of emergencies.

Many dental specialists, even with whatever qualifications they possess, feel CPCR training may not be applicable to them, as they may not be directly involved with medical issues. Some dentists even boast that no emergency ever happened in their clinic, even during their practice of 20 to 30 years.

The authors felt that the dental surgeon can be in a very awkward situation if an emergency arises while performing dental procedures and minor surgeries in a small set- up in the nook and corner of India. Emergencies may happen in the absence of any infrastructure for resuscitation; monitors, oxygen supply, and the nearest emergency-competent hospital may be far away. One must think of a situation that may arise in one's busy practice in a remote area with neither the facility for resuscitation in the clinic nor quick access to emergency care at a hospital nearby. It will be devastating for the doctor or dentist, the patient, and their family if a death occurs in circumstances without immediate assistance. At this moment of crisis, the dental specialist would feel that the availability of resuscitation drugs and equipment in a clinic was mandatory and that training emergencies and CPCR probably would have saved the patient.

When medical negligence becomes an issue in a court of law, what is expected from a dentist who faces a medical emergency is a "reasonable standard of care" under the circumstances. So, if dentist has made some attempt to revive the patient by using whatever emergency equipment was available in the clinic, gross negligence would not be attributed to the dentist. The defense attorney can present such an argument on behalf of the dentist, which the court is often prepared to accept.

3.4.1 CPCR Training

The training may be given in two ways: basic and advanced. [1]

Basic and advanced courses
A basic certificate course is intended for all health professionals, including dentists, and addresses the primary emergency care for the patient in case of a collapse in a dental chair or any place of treatment or public place.

This is normally done as daylong training, for an affordable fee, by many professional centres and institutions that are accredited to provide basic and advanced training to all health professionals. The course involves lectures and discussions on recent advances in CPCR and hands-on, practical training in manikins and emergency drug usage.

Though certain centres provide courses that are credentialed by the American Heart Association (AHA), it is not mandatory unless one is planning to go to the USA or Europe for their future career.

The *advanced course* is taken after the basic skill course for emergencies. Usually, this will be done by medical and dental professionals who are involved in the everyday practice of medical as well as surgical management. This is a 3-day training program with an emphasis on emergency situation identification, IV cannulation, ECG monitoring, CPCR training, including the use of a defibrillator (AED), and, medical drug management in different emergency situations. With this training, one would be able to perform a credible CPCR for primary emergencies in any situation, with access to equipment for resuscitation and necessary drugs. Refresher courses are recommended as protocols for emergency management, based on recent changes that facilitate optimal management of emergency situations. It is also possible that dentists can get trained to become trainers by taking special courses on this subject.

One should check the status of all resuscitation equipment and emergency drugs in their dental clinic regularly and be vigilant about the expiry dates of drugs and materials used in emergency situations. Expired drugs can produce embarrassing issues that may compromise the credibility of the clinic. Often, many drugs have similar-sounding names, which can lead to serious errors and mishaps during emergencies. The author recalls an occasion when ketamine was administered instead of ketoroloc, which led to a life-threatening emergency.[1]

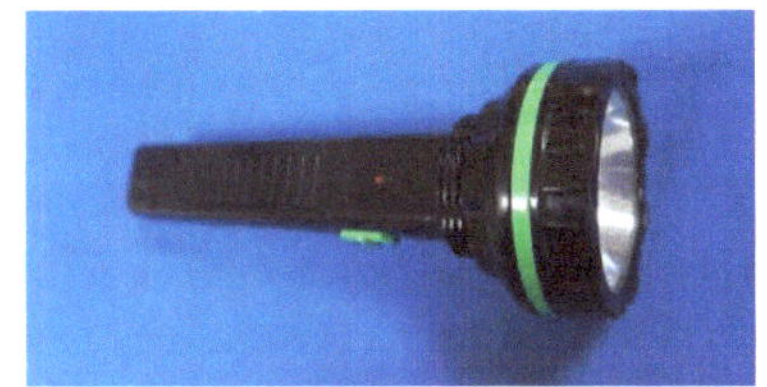

Figure 3.1 (c): Torch (battery)

3.5 Emergency Equipments

Figure 3.1 (a)-(j)

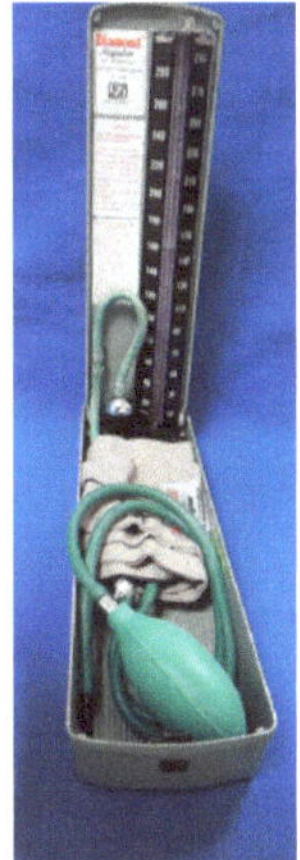

Figure 3.1 (a): BP apparatus

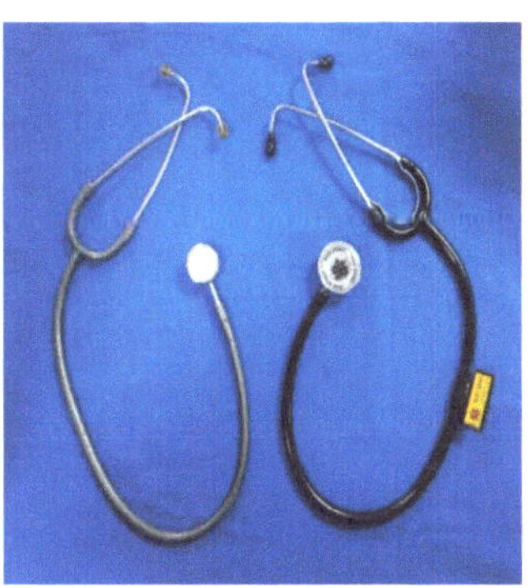

Figure 3.1 (b): Paediatric and Adult Stethoscope

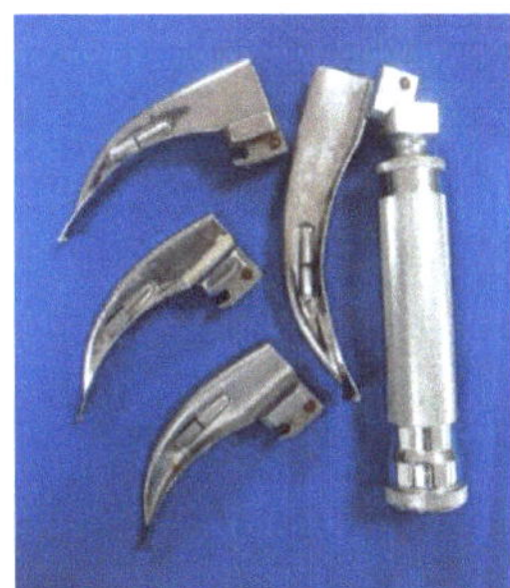

Figure 3.1 (d): Larynoscope

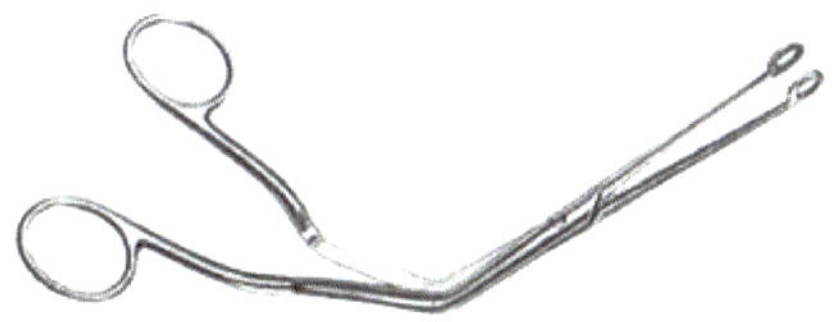

Figure 3.1 (e): Magill's intubating forcep

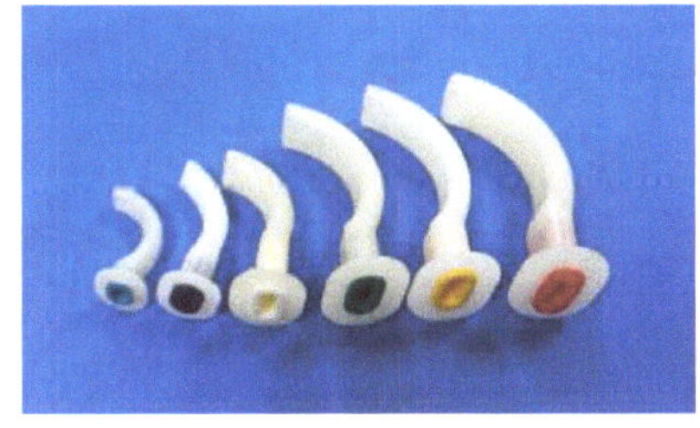

Figure 3.1 (f): Water's oropharyngeal air way

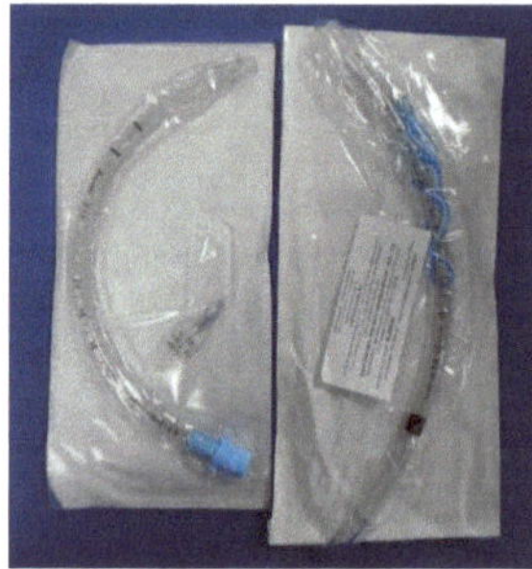

Figure 3.1 (g): Endotracheal tubes

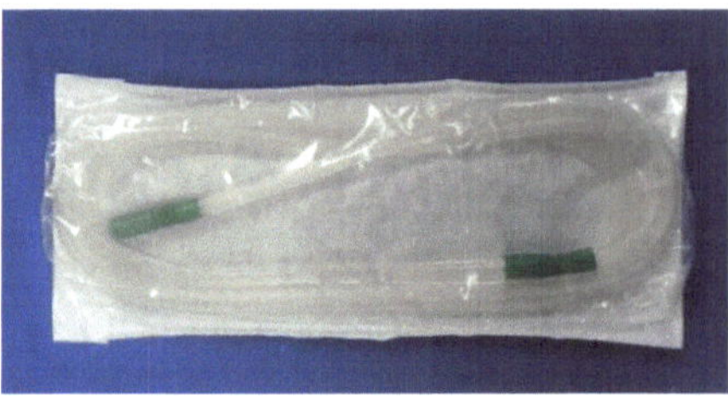

Figure 3.1 (j): Suction catheters

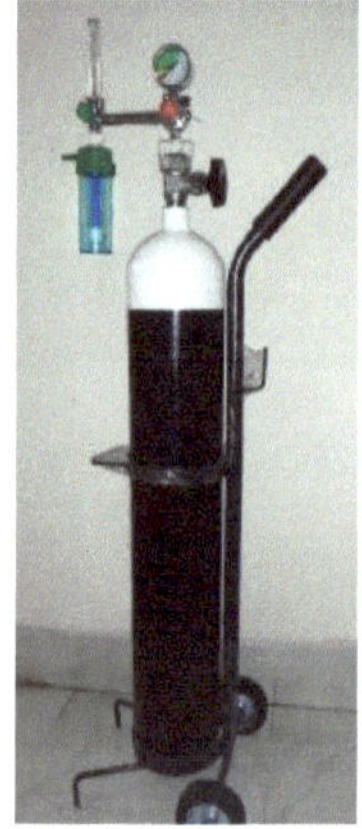

Figure 3.1 (h): O2 cylinder with flow meter and humidifier

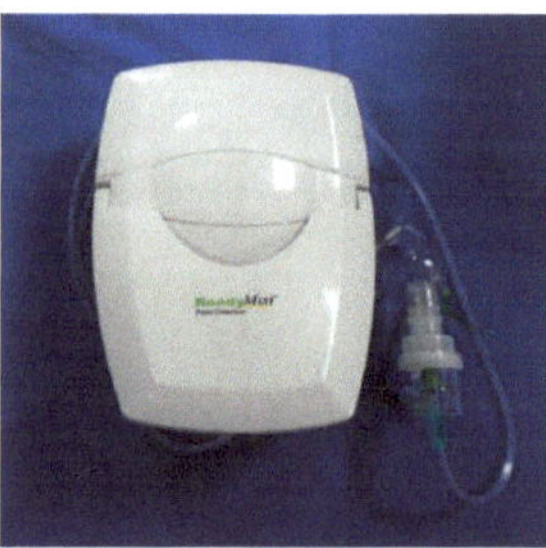

Figure 3.1 (i): Nebulizer

3.6 Emergency Drugs

Emergency Drugs[2]

Adrenaline IP 1:1000 inj.

Atropine sulfate inj.

Sodium hydrocortisone succinate inj.

Dextrose 25% & 50% inj.

Aminophylline inj.

Dopamine inj.

Diazepam, Midazolam

Fortwin inj.

Sodium Bicarbonate inj.

Tab Nitroglycerine

Inj Nitroglycerine

Phenergan / Avil tab/ inj.

Promethazine (Perinorm)

Water for injection

Frusemide (Lasix) inj.

Aerosol spray epinephrine, salbutamol

IV fluids dextrose 5%, Ringer lactate, Normal saline.

IV set

Scalp vein set

IV cannula

Disposable syringes with needles 2 ml, 5 ml, and 10 ml.

Name of the drug	Dose	Indications/uses
1. Atropine sulphate (Anticholinergic)	0.6 mg IM/IV	1. Vasovagal shock. 2. Prevention of bradycardia 3. Preanaesthetic medication. 4. To reduce salivary secretions.
2. Adrenaline tartarate 1:1000	0.5-1.0 mg. IV/SC or intracardiac, to be repeated every five minutes	1. Cardiac arrest. 2. Anaphylactic shock. 3. Severe laryngobroncheal spasm
3. Dexamethasone	4-20 mg of IM or IV 05-50 mg. per day orally	1. Cereberal edema. 2. Allergic conditions. 3. Anti inflammatory 4. Shock 5. Immunosupression
4. Sodium hydrocortisone sodium succinate/ hemisuccinate (short acting glucocorticoid).	100 mg IM/IV Stat; may be repeated once or twice	1. Shock 2. Status asthamaticus 3. Acute adrenal insufficiency 4. Anaphylactic reaction. 5 Allergic reaction.
5. Pheniramine maleate TN- avil	Orally-25-50 mg tabs. 25 mg 1 tid 50 mg 1 bid ampule- 1-2 ml IM 12 hrly Vial 1-2 ml IM 12 hrly	1. Allergic reactions. 2. Rigors. 3. Sedative. 4. Anaphylactic shock. 5. Angioneurotic edema.
6. Promethazine hydrochloride.	Orally, 10 mg, 2 mg tabs. Injection 2ml.	1. Allergy 2. Nausea.
7. Diazepam (benzodiazepine derivative. Note: - it should not be mixed with other drugs for IV infusion.	Orally 5-40 mg. Injection 10 mg, 3-4 times IV	1. Anti-anxiety. 2. In acute muscle spasm. 3. Spastic neurological disease. 4. Tetanus. 5. Electroconsulsive therapy. 6. Orthopaedic manipulation.
8. Deriphylline (bronchodilator). Etophylline 169.4 mg, Theophylline 50.6 mg, per 2ml injection.	2-4 ml. Upto 2-3 times daily IV. (2ml in one minute IM & SC also; as a combined injection with dextrose).	1. Bronchial asthma. 2. Cardiac insufficiency. 3. Central respiratory disorder 4. Renal & cardiac edema.
9. Aminophylline (methylxanthine)	250-500 mg. diluted in 20-50 ml. of 5% dextrose; infuse IV over 20-30 minutes' repeat as required.	1. Status asthmaticus.
10. Mephenteramine (adrenergic drug).	Orally 10-20 mg. tabs; or IM or IV (to prepare IV drip 2 vials of 30 mg. each are added to 500 ml of 5% dextrose sol.)	1. Shock in myocardial infarction 2. Hypotension due to spinal anesthesia. 3. Other hypotensive states.
11. Dopamine (adrenergic alfa & beta agonist)	0.2–1.0 mg per minute. IV	1. Shock cardiogenic 2. Severe congestive heart failure.

Name of the drug	Dose	Indications/uses
12. Frusemide. TN- Lasix	Orally, 40 mg tabs. In edema 20-80 mg. Single dose daily	1. Edema in congestive heart failure. 2. Hepatic or renal disease. 3. Toxaemia of pregnancy. 4. Mild and moderate hypertension. 5. Cereberal edema.
13. Isosorbide dinitrate TN- Sorbitrate.	Sub-lingual 5-10 mg. for immediate action, orally 5-10 mg six hourly.	1. Angina pectoris.
14. Pentazocin TN-Fortwin	Orally 50-100 mg tabs 30-60 mg IM/SC	1. Moderate to severe pain after surgery. 2. Trauma, colic, burns. 3. Pre-anaesthetic medications.
15. Metoclopramide. TN- Perinorm. (more effective if combined with H2 blocker)	25-50 mg IM orally, 5-10 mg thrice daily.	1. Premedication 2. Migraine. 3. Antiemetic.
16. Ringer lactate	1- 2 pint IV. (based on the body weight)	1. Dehydration 2. Burns.
17. Dextrose ampule 25-50%	1-2 amp IV.	Hypoglycemia/Hypoglycemic shock
18. Haemaccel (plasma expander)	1 pint IV.	Hypovolemic shock.
19. Sodabicarb	1ml mole/kg. body weight 50% of dose repeated every 10-15 min. (IV)	Metabolic acidosis.
20. Spirit of ammonia	1 drop in nose	Reflex stimulation in fainting or hysteria.
21. Normal saline	1 -2 pint (based on the body weight) IV	1. Hypoosmolality. 2. Vehicle for intravenous drug administration.
22. Oxygen	3-5lit/min.	1. Hypoxia 2. Shock 3. Cardiorespiratory failure.
23. Pethidine	50 mg IM	1. Severe pain. 2. Pre-anaesthetic medication.

3.7 Look-alike Medications

When an emergency happens in a clinic, at least one person should be responsible for the maintenance of medications, writing on a notepad what drugs have been given and the dose administered, and also transferring the information to a higher centre if the patient is shifted.

Occasionally, look-alike medications in ampoules can be mistakenly given, leading to catastrophic outcomes rather than bringing the patient out of danger. The way to avoid this is to be careful when labelling each medication in the drug tray and have a clear chart in the clinic for easy application.

The following is an example of "look-alike packaging" from around the world. Most of these are still in clinical circulation, exposing patients to the risks. **(Figure 3.2)**

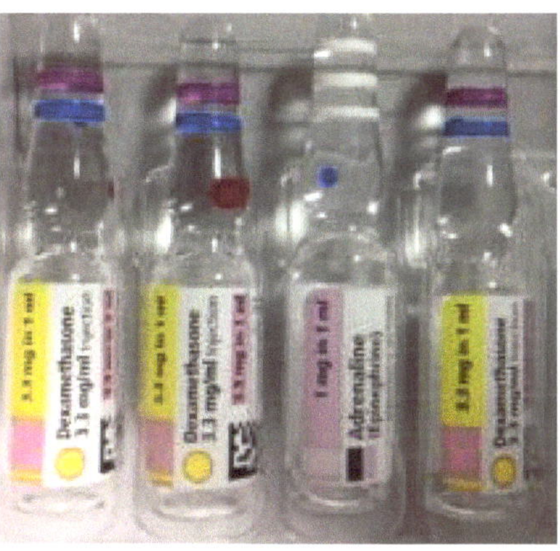

Figure 3.2: Look alike medications

References:

1. Resuscitation Council UK. Medical emergencies and resuscitation - standards for clinical practice and training for dental practitioners and dental care professionals in general dental practice. London: Resuscitation Council UK, 2011.
2. Malamed SF. Handbook of local anesthesia-e-book. Elsevier health sciences; 2019 Mar 28.

Physical Injury and Forensic Examination

4.1 Introduction

Physical injury in the context of forensic medicine has been defined as the: "damage to any part of the body due to the deliberate or accidental application of mechanical or another traumatic agent".

This chapter focuses on the evaluation of physical assaults committed against people who have been taken to emergency care, as well as the evaluation and documentation of wounds or injuries.

Along with professionals from emergency medicine department, the maxillofacial surgeon could be among the first doctors to examine such a patient and document the signs of damage. Evaluation and documentation serve to help prove the source of a wound or damage, which is frequently a point of contention in legal proceedings. Any physician or dentist should be able to do these two tasks.

In the author's experience, interpretation of the injury is crucial, as are the records of the primary surgery performed, the number of sutures applied, and the state of the wounds, whether clean or with ragged edges. All such information plays out in front of the law. In court, a cross-examining person can counter our argument about the use of alleged instruments vs. the fall theory. A thorough and proper documentation of the details of the examination and reporting is absolutely important.

Given that there may be several elements involved in such interpretation, it is usually best left to professionals with forensic knowledge to interpret the underlying causes of wounds and injuries. It is crucial that the descriptions are clear to everyone since interpreting wounds and injuries may be done by looking at documentation, such as written explanations, body chart mapping, or images.

The first examination and evaluation may have been performed in many cases only for therapeutic reasons, and it might be weeks or months before the forensic relevance of the injuries is understood. Examining the notes written by the physician later, potentially in court, may uncover severe errors that could seriously jeopardize the legal procedures as well as the reputation of the particular doctor and the profession as a whole. Non-specialist doctors may come across injured patients, and the treatment may cause conflict during legal processes.

4.2 Assessment and Documentation

A thorough history, a proper physical examination, and contemporaneous, clear documentation of the results are all necessary for injury evaluation and analysis. Additional doctors, legal counsel, and the courts may evaluate such material (either notes, body charts, or computer information). The person being examined should be asked for their consent before beginning the examination and before producing a medical report as a result. Additionally, it should be kept in mind that frivolous or vexatious claims of assault are possible, and the person reviewing the case ought to recognize that false accusations and counter-allegations sometimes happen, sometimes only becoming apparent in hindsight. [1]

4.2.1 Key Factors in the Examination

The important elements listed in **Table 1** should be considered when examining anyone who has been presented with maxillofacial injuries and, if applicable, should be identified when the injured person's history is obtained.

Documenting the alleged timing of the injury's occurrence is crucial. Because injuries heal over time, how they manifest after an assault depends on the passage of time. Several injuries to various body parts are possible. Each component should be thoroughly examined.

If recognized, note the victim's and attacker's handedness (left, right, or both), since this might influence how damage causation is interpreted. Witnesses may provide conflicting versions of what happened; it is the forensic doctor's job to help the court determine which version is accurate. It is necessary to evaluate the impact that drugs, alcohol, or both might have on each instance, given that these narratives may also be affected by these substances.

Since every specific kind of weapon can create distinguishable injuries, knowing the type that was used might be crucial when assessing injuries. It is important to examine the type of clothing worn (such as armless vests or long-sleeved shirts). All these characteristics should be considered when evaluating any person who has been taken to A&E for injuries. Some of these characteristics may become significant as the examination goes on or when further accounts of any attack are provided. [1,2]

Table 1: Potentially relevant factors to be determined from history

SL. No.	Relevant factors to be determined from history
1.	How was the injury sustained?
2.	Weapon or weapons used (is it [are they] still available?)
3.	What time was the injury sustained?
4.	Has the injury been treated?
5.	Pre-existing illnesses (e.g., skin disease).
6.	Regular physical activity (e.g., contact sports).
7.	Regular medication (e.g., anticoagulants, steroids).
8.	Handedness of victim and suspect.
9.	Use of drugs and alcohol.
10.	Clothing worn.

Annotated pro-forma diagrams, handwritten notes, and photographs are all acceptable forms of injury documentation. A body chart and note system are depicted in one type in **Figure 4.1.**

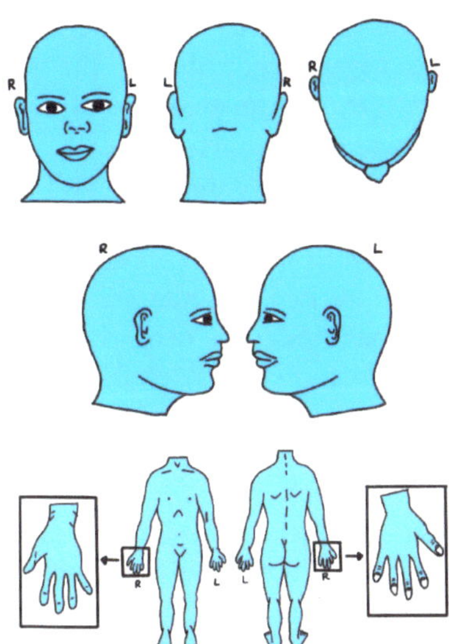

Figure 4.1: Body chart and note system

The features of each injury are listed in **Table 2** and may be required for proper documentation.

Table 2: Potentially relevant information required when assessing injuries

SL. No.	Details to be recorded when assessing injuries
1.	Location (anatomical—measure distance from landmarks)
2.	Type (e.g., bruise, cut, or abrasion)
3.	Size (use metric values)
4.	Shape
5.	Pain
6.	Causation
7.	Color
8.	Tenderness
9.	Orientation
10.	Stiffness
11.	Age
12.	Time
13.	Transientness (of injury)
14.	Handedness

It is now acceptable to use digital photos to record an injury, but the electronic evidence must be accompanied by concurrent written and hand-drawn notes. Make sure that each injury is covered by the narrative given at the time of inspection.

At that point, you should query any injuries that don't match the patient's or a family member's description. People who suffer injuries in fights or other violent situations frequently are simply unaware of the origin of numerous injury locations. Re-examining injuries 24–48 hours later to assess how they change, whether bruises have emerged, or whether other sites of injury are obvious may be helpful (especially with blunt impact). Photography and inspection done before and after therapy might be helpful.

4.3 Types of Injury

Anyone participating in injury assessment should be aware of the variety of terminology that might be used to describe various injuries. In order to guarantee that the basis of any given injury is accurately, repeatedly, and explicitly stated in note form using established words of categorization, every doctor should have their own method.

The most frequent reasons why medical evidence on injuries given in court is disputed are the use of a complex array of phrases by doctors and an improper or erroneous description of a wound. For instance, calling an incision a "laceration" when it was actually a clean-cut wound brought on by a bladed weapon, such as knife.

Therefore, it is essential to employ a standard nomenclature when describing injuries for medico-legal purposes. The categorization that follows is precise and simple, and most apparent injuries will fall into one of the classes listed in **Table 3**.

Table 3: Classification of Injuries

Wheals and erythema (reddening)	Bruises (contusion or ecchymosis)
Hematoma	Petechiae
Abrasions	Scratches
(grazes)	Point abrasion
Scuff/brush abrasions	Incisions
Lacerations	Chop
Slash	Firearms
Stab wounds	Bites

The indicators or indications of a blunt force hit can vary, and the damage they cause depends on a number of variables, including force, position, and striking surface. These injuries might include "no visible evidence" of harm, discomfort, or soreness at the area of contact, swelling, reddening, abrasions, bruises, cuts (lacerations), and shattered bones. Each type of damage might occur on its own or in combination. Where the impacting object initially makes contact with the body, these wounds are evident.

After some time, bruises may move away from the place of contact due to gravity. The impact point may clearly be identified by abrasions. In rare circumstances, damage patterns might reveal if a specific hitting object was present. According to the amount of force used, blunt impact injuries can be classified as mild, mild/moderate, moderate, moderate/severe, or severe.

Sharp injuries are those brought on by objects with cutting edges, such as glass, knives, or scissors. The wounds might be (i) incised, where the cutting edge runs perpendicular to the skin's surface, slicing through skin and deeper anatomical tissues, or (ii) stabbed, when the sharp edge penetrates the skin into deeper structures. In contrast to stab wounds, which are often deeper than they are wide, incised wounds are typically longer than they are deep. Because a sharp, pointed item may easily puncture important tissues, such as neck vessels, the forces necessary to create such injuries and their effects vary. Special kinds of cutting wounds included those caused by slash or chop wounds from tools like machetes.[3]

Numerous hits may result in immediate discomfort and agony that pass quickly, as well as soreness that may last for hours or days without showing any obvious signs of damage. The layperson must be mindful that an assault or injury does not necessarily go uninjured just because there are no obvious signs of it.

After an injury, such as a slap, scrape, or punch, which may go unnoticed in a few hours, such as a bruise or erythema, early vasodilatation and local release of vasoactive peptides also induce wounds and erythema. The triple reaction's traditional characteristics are present, yet no particular tissue damage is caused. As a result, unlike bruising, which will still be visible after 24 hours or more, an initial reddening coupled with discomfort and the potential future development of local swelling may be observed immediately.[1]

4.3.1 Size and Shape of the Injury

The size of a wound is possibly the most commonly forgotten item in medical records, despite the fact that it may be the easiest measurement to calculate.

It must be measured in centimeters or millimeters and recorded using calipers or a ruler. Since measurements presented in imperial units may be easier for some individuals to understand, the comparable size of an injury in inches may also be included. The shape of the wound should also be noted; basic terms, such as "circular," "triangular," "V-shaped," or "crescent-shaped," work best to express this feature; however, if the shape of the wound is intricate or irregular, it might be easier to put this data on a body chart. Even though it can occasionally be difficult to accurately assess it in a living person, the depth of a wound may also exist.

4.3.2 Position of the Injury

The best method of pinpointing the location of an injury is to use fixed anatomical landmarks. On the head, one can use the eyes, ears, nose, and mouth; on the neck, the prominence of the thyroid cartilage and the sternocleidomastoid muscles can be used; and on the trunk, the nipples, umbilicus, and bony prominences can be used as points of reference. The advantages of using simple anatomical diagrams and body charts for locating the injury are self-evident. It is a simple process to record the position of an injury accurately, yet when medical records are reviewed, it is both surprising and disappointing to find only a vague indication of location.

4.3.3 Ageing Injuries

One of the most often asked about and contested topics in forensic medicine, a specialist in forensics will set aside a specified amount of time or time period to examine how an injury was caused. The process of healing relies on a number of variables, such as the injury site, the force used, the degree of tissue damage, infection, therapy, etc. As a result, it is very challenging and imprecise to determine the age of a wound.

After an injury, blood diffuses closer to the skin's surface, making bruises more visible for a few hours or even days. An older, more superficial lesion may occasionally be mistaken for a recent significant bruising. Bruises fade over a period of days to weeks; how long it takes depends on the size of the bruise. Depending on the examiner's perception of colour, a bruise may be blue, mauve, purple, brown, green, yellow, or all variations of these colors and tones.

Red, blue, purple, or black bruises may emerge at any time from the start of bruising until resolution as much as 21 days as per the only substantial study that looked at the colour evolution of bruises. Yellow bruises, on the other hand, were shown to be older than eighteen hours. The color of bruises and the evolution and shift in colour patterns cannot be used to time the damage, with the unusual exception of a yellow bruise that may be considered to be older than eighteen hours.

It should be made clear that since the color measurements are inaccurate, estimating the age of the bruise color images is likewise erratic and shouldn't be depended upon. Another study that recently found significant variation among observers in color matching when performed in vivo and in digital reproductions has verified this. Only other precise evidence, such as color witnessed strike, may accurately pinpoint when a bruise occurred. [4]

Abrasions acquired during life often have a reddish-brown color and release blood and serum, which solidify to create a scab. This scab forms over many days until it separates to reveal a pink, often undamaged surface. While incisions, the margins of which may be in opposition, tend to heal in a few days, while some may leave severe scarring. Lacerations often heal with scarring over a number of days or weeks without medical intervention.

4.3.4 Transient Lesions

Despite being commonly brought on by trauma, swelling, redness, and pain are not always indicative of damage. Although it's crucial to note whether these characteristics are present, it's also necessary to keep in mind that these lesions might potentially have non-traumatic origins, such as eczema, dermatitis, or impetigo. Red markings denoting an apparent injury, such as an impression of a hand on a slapped face, should be recorded as soon as possible because such pictures may vanish in about an hour and leave no lasting imprints.

References:

1. Singh V, Malkunje L, Mohammad S, Singh N, Dhasmana S, Das SK. The maxillofacial injuries: A study. Natl J Maxillofac Surg. 2012 Jul;3(2):166-71. doi: 10.4103/0975-5950.111372.

2. Gassner R, Tuli T, Hächl O, Rudisch A, Ulmer H. Cranio-maxillofacial trauma: a 10 year review of 9,543 cases with 21,067 injuries. J Craniomaxillofac Surg. 2003 Feb;31(1):51-61. doi: 10.1016/s1010-5182(02)00168-3.

3. Lopes Sá CD, Silva PB, Correia AM, Soares EC, Bezerra TP, Melo RB, Bitú HS, Costa FW. Maxillofacial and dental-related injuries from a Brazilian forensic science institute: Victims and perpetrators characteristics and associated risk factors. J Clin Exp Dent. 2020 Aug 1;12(8):e736-e744. doi: 10.4317/jced.56637.

4. Chen JY, Wang WC, Chen YK, Lin LM. A retrospective study of trauma-associated oral and maxillofacial lesions in a population from southern Taiwan. J Appl Oral Sci. 2010 Jan-Feb;18(1):5-9. doi: 10.1590/s1678-77572010000100003.

Assessment of Injury to the Dentofacial Region for Issuing Wound Certificate, Police Intimation and Documentation in Accident Register

5.1 Introduction

Physical injury in the context of forensic medicine is defined as the "damage to any part of the body due to the deliberate or accidental application of mechanical or another traumatic agent".

All injuries sustained due to road traffic accidents, interpersonal violence, or by any means that have a medicolegal connotation must be recorded as per the requirements of the law. This is to ensure that the evidence can be used to establish the nature and extent of injury by a court of law or by any administration of justice or social welfare scheme (disability), etc.

Injuries presenting to the emergency room or hospital must be assessed through meticulous history-taking and evaluation of the injuries to ascertain if there are medico-legal implications. Dentists and oral and maxillofacial surgeons are often called upon to assess injuries in their respective regions.

5.1.1 Wound Certificate

After making benchmark identification of the patient by name, address, and permanent identifying points (like moles, scars, etc.), the details of the accident have to be entered and recorded in the appropriate form in the manner described by the accompanying person or the patient, who has to be identified. In the absence of credible evidence, all details of the nature of the accident have to be entered as '**alleged**'. For example, '*alleged assault* by known or unknown persons or alleged road traffic accident while travelling on a two-wheeler' etc. Details such as the place and registration number of injuries to vehicles involved and the names of persons involved should be clearly mentioned.

The nature, size, and site of the injuries must be clearly described using standard accepted terms described later. The injuries can be classified as grievous or simple, based on the schema described below. For example, a maxillofacial surgeon attending to injuries to a facial injury will need to describe fractures, if any, degree of displacement, soft tissue injuries of the region, injury to teeth, including loss of teeth, etc. In the author's experience, many cases of denial of insurance claims have been reported due to the failure to prevent tooth loss from accidents in future rehabilitation. The wound certificate must be signed by the attending specialists with the official seal of the doctors, including their registration numbers. **(Figure 5.1)**

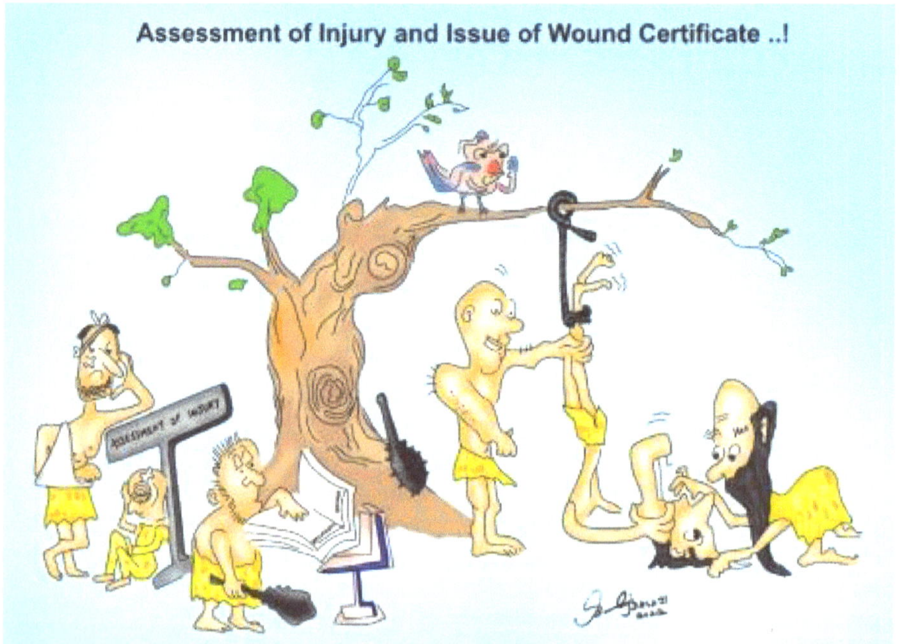

Figure 5.1: Assessment of injury and issue of wound certificate

5.1.2 Accident Register (AR)

Accident registers are maintained in all emergency rooms, and they should be filled out in the same manner, explaining all the details. A police intimation is made by the casualty doctor or by the treating surgeon or physician to the station of jurisdiction. They will rely on the accident registration and personal inquiry to prepare the **Mahzar** (petition) and register a **First Information Report** (**FIR**) if it is a medical-legal case. Police reports from the police officials made at the site of the accident may also be collated into the report.

Emergency management is the first priority:

In case any emergency treatment is required to stabilize the patient, it will be the first priority of the treating doctor, and it takes precedence over all formalities, including police intimation and even billing or informed consent. This has been established by several Supreme Court rulings, starting with Paramananda Katara vs. Union of India (1989) and others. Inability to identify the patient, medico-legal considerations, inability to pay, etc. are not reasons for not instituting emergency care to stabilize the patient.

5.1.3 Treatment Certificate

Treatment certificate issued by the treating doctor must identify the patient, cause, time, and nature of the injury. The treatment details should indicate the timeline, anaesthesia, surgical or medical procedure, and outcome. It should also mention the post-operative sequelae, including rehabilitation, and the anticipated time when the patient will be fit for work, study, or normal activity.

Dentists and Maxillofacial surgeons as expert witnesses
Maxillofacial surgeons and dentists are frequently asked to provide testimony in criminal and civil trials. A dentist has to be knowledgeable about the topic when asked to provide testimony in the context of forensic evidence. [1] Although forensic dentistry has been utilised, it will only be briefly discussed in this book in an entirely separate section. In India, forensic dentistry has been employed in a number of high-profile cases, the most well-known of which is the assassination of former Prime Minister Rajiv Gandhi.

Dental surgeons are often called up in other, more common situations as well:
1.   A disability assessment following dental or maxillofacial injuries

2.   For feedback on the practices used by other medical professionals or dentists in situations of suspected carelessness.

As was covered previously in the chapter, *summons* is issued for witnesses who are experts. The dentist has to appear in court at the scheduled time. He may be questioned about the type of injury and the extent of the handicap by the attorneys for the prosecution, the defense, or the insurance company. The dentist must express his views unequivocally and concisely and should avoid making commitments to issues he is unsure of. When testifying, he will be provided a copy of any wound certificates that the dentist provided for his reference. Just the facts must be stated by the witness. He is unlikely to be asked to research the relevant legal issues. For instance, losing teeth, breaking teeth, etc. He is permitted to honestly respond to any further inquiries on the same. [1]

For dental and maxillofacial impairment, there are currently no defined disability criteria in India. The standards for oral and maxillofacial impairments and abnormalities are currently being developed by the Association of Oral and Maxillofacial Surgeons. Dentists might utilize the somewhat scanty reference from "The Manual for Permanent Disability," published in 1981 by the CGHS, WHO, and AIIMS. The Mc Brides disability criterion and the American Association of Oral and Maxillofacial Surgeons' standards (which might not be very applicable to our group) are further sources of information. A dentist, however, can determine if the damage is severe or not. He could go into further detail about the specific impairment that the law might bring about.

A few examples of *grievous injuries* are as follows:

1. Tooth loss.
2. Tooth fracture.
3. Tooth avulsion.
4. Tooth's vitality testis negative.
5. Fracture involving facial bone
6. Soft tissue loss and significant scarring.
7. Neurological impairment (sensory or motor)

Based on a variety of Indian and international standards, the author has suggested suggestions for disabilities and deformities. This could be approved after careful consideration. It is also argued why exactly a criterion should exist.

5.2 Quantification of Dento-facial Disability or Deformity

A Proposal (George Paul and Sam Thomas, 2003)

The fundamental elements of human existence are form and function. This equilibrium is disrupted by impairment and deformity. Deformity or disability can be inherited or acquired. Authorities have a social obligation to lessen these ailments by fostering conditions that will allow for their reintegration into regular social life. The majority of welfare states offer assistance to people with disabilities.

Injuries, interpersonal aggression, and iatrogenic factors can all result in disability. These scenarios have legal ramifications and frequently call for payment of some kind. The handicap must be quantified in order to compute compensation and benefits.

Orthopaedic impairments have been measured and calibrated in both civilian and military life. The same goes for various impairments that involve locomotor, neurological, visual, and hearing deficits. However, none of these quantification charts fully cover the maxillofacial area.

Because there are two separate criteria to be evaluated—disability and deformity—[2] quantification of the maxillofacial area is distinct. Deformity is mostly a matter of opinion, making any compensation for it arbitrary, whereas disability can be quantified more easily. The deformity of the face, however, cannot be disregarded, so an effort is made to construct a wide dimension in which it may be evaluated.

5.2.1 Review of Quantification Criteria

Orthopaedic disability quantification is widely established and has been used for social advantages, rehabilitation, support, and percentage reservations in the placement of handicapped individuals in the labor market. [2] Additionally, it has been used for legal and insurance settlements resulting from mishaps, violent crimes, and occupational illnesses. The Canadian Army created the Phulhems profile as early as 1943. Up until 1980, India used the McBrides criterion as the standard. It was commonly acknowledged for injuries to the teeth and tooth loss, and it did include some areas of the maxillofacial region. In India, the *"Manual for Doctors to Evaluate Permanent Physical Impairment"* (1981) took on the role of the McBrides criterion (1955). However, the face is only given a small portion of a chapter—one half—and only receives about 30 points, making the damage and handicap of the face relatively vaguely and weakly described. The 45 advisors on the advisory committee did not include a single Maxillofacial surgeon.

There are several references accessible in the fields of orthopaedics and rehabilitation after injury. Different facets of both lower and upper extremity impairments were examined by Kessler (1970). Through a series of queries that determine the durability of the deficiency, the American Academy of Orthopaedic Surgeons Manual (1966) explores the idea of an irreversible impairment. The Govt. of India notification (1986) addresses hearing and speech impairments as well as locomotor and vision disorders. It suggests using Kessler's formula as a broad rule of thumb. Notably, the Government of Tamil Nadu's statement from 1974 contains the only other Indian guidelines for the Maxillofacial region and addresses total facial deformity. It just grants a 50% penalty for overall facial deformity. There are no numbers broken down by deformity type or degree.

Guidelines for evaluating Maxillofacial injuries and disabilities have been provided by the American Medical Association and the American Association of Oral and Maxillofacial Surgeons. To meet the demands of our people, they must, however, be modified.

Two key sources were used by the writers when conducting this evaluation.

1. Sabapathy vinayagam Ramar's Objective Evaluation of Impairment and Ability in Locomotor Handicapped a top-notch resource on physical therapy and rehabilitation.

2. The American Association of Oral and Maxillofacial Regions published Guidelines for the Evaluation of Impairment of the Oral and Maxillofacial Regions.

To come up with the suggestions, the writers adjusted the guidelines from the sources mentioned above.

The overall goal of the activity was to develop quantitative criteria for the maxillofacial region's limitations and deformities while taking into account the unique characteristics of the issues faced in India. Additionally, it tries to make the proportions provided simpler by getting rid of complicated factors.

The evaluation takes the stance that the face should receive a 100% score, with deformity receiving 50% and impairment receiving 50%. Since doing so would drastically diminish the severity of the impairment and negate the aim of the exercise, it does not attempt to analyse face impairment as a component of overall impairment. Take into account a scenario where 100% must be allocated to the circulatory, digestive, neurological, and locomotor systems in addition to sexual, hepatic, renal, endocrine, and metabolic dysfunctions. Additional distribution among the visual, auditory, etc. will undoubtedly reduce any assistance in putting value on the face.

Additionally, the examination has removed the need to consider factors that might have changed the award percentages, such as age, sex, and employment. These will fall within the purview of governmental organisations, the judicial system, or insurance representatives.

According to standards defined within the scope of the 100% for the face, evenly distributed across the primary frameworks and functions, the criteria merely provide a statement of handicap or deformity. The sum of them should, using the formula, not exceed one hundred.

$$A + B \frac{(100 - A)}{100}$$

where A denotes the higher value and B denotes the lower value.

5.2.2 Definitions

Based on Govt. of India Gazette Part I, Section 1 No. 4-2/83, HW III Ministry of Welfare, 1986.8

Impairment is defined as any loss or abnormality of psychological, physiological, or anatomical structure or function.

Disability: WHO defines disability in the context of health experience as any restriction or lack (resulting from an impairment) of ability to perform an activity in the manner (or) within the range considered normal for a human being.

Deformity: facial disfigurement involving soft and hard tissues arising from multiple genetic factors, environmental influences, acquired defects, neoplastic processes, and trauma.

Recommended Quantification for the Dentofacial Region

Areas of Deformity Evaluation – Hard Tissues:

A. Loss of Teeth:

Anteriors	Deformity / Disability
All anterior (upper and lower):	25%
Between 8 to 11:	20%
Between 4 to 7:	15%
Between 2 to 3:	10%
One tooth:	05%

Although these impairments and abnormalities may be corrected, they warrant the higher percentile since artificial teeth aren't considered to be as strong and functional as real teeth. Even when prostheses are provided, orthopedic abnormalities are assessed.

Posteriors	Disability
Including premolars but excluding third molars.	
All posteriors (16 teeth):	25%
Between 10 to 14:	20%
Between 6 to 9:	15%
Between 2 to 5:	10%
Occlusal discrepancy:	10%-20%
Single tooth:	05%

Areas of Deformity Evaluation – Hard Tissues:

Tooth loss brought on by developing dental disease (such as periodontitis or caries) is not taken into account. The dental surgeon must do an evaluation based on the state of the teeth that remain or previous data.

B. Loss of Bone   Disability / Deformity%

Significant loss of bone causing

Deformity/Disability: 10%-25%

Small bony fragment: 5%

C. Malunited Facial Bones: (Depending on extent of Disability / Deformity)

Malunited facial bones   10%-20%

- Occlusion to be combined whenever affected.

This is only a partial quantification, and the surgeon will need to judge it based on how much handicap or deformity the malunion has created.

D. Orbital Deformity (excluding visual field assessment)

Subjective evaluation based on:

Bony orbit: 5%-10%

Soft tissue (e.g.) ectropion, scar etc.:   5%-10%

Composite deformities including

Telecanthus etc.:   15%-25%

Areas of Deformity Evaluation – Soft Tissue:

A. Soft Tissue – Non-reversible

Single linear scar: 5%

Multiple or deforming scars

Including keloids: 10%-30%

Significant loss of soft tissue

E.g. Loss of nose, ear, lips etc.:   20%-50%

B. Facial Sensory Impairment (RAMAR)

Face has 34% sensory innervations of whole body.

Ophthalmic: 8%

Maxillary: 8%

Mandibular: 8%

Tongue: 10%

C. Impairment Rate for Mouth Opening (RAMAR)

Impairment rate for inter incisor distance of 4 cms: 0%

Impairment rate for inter incisor distance of 3 cms: 10%

Impairment rate for inter incisor distance of 2 cms: 20%

Impairment rate for inter incisor distance of 1 cm: 30%

Impairment rate for inter incisor distance of 0 cm: 50%

Areas of Deformity Evaluation – Soft Tissue:

D. Motor Disability (RAMAR)

Jaw muscles (masticatory):   5% right side, 5% left side

Tongue muscles: 15% either side.

E. Facial Nerve Impairment

Single branch: 05%

Five branches: 25%

Zygomaticotemporal: 10%

Bilateral problems are not addressed.

F. Disfigurement criteria (AAOMS and AMA guidelines 1997 and 2002)

Class 1-(0-5%) Disorder of cutaneous structure e.g. visible scars

Class 2- (5-10%) loss of supporting structure with or without cutaneous disorder e.g. depressed cheek and nose.

Class 3- (10-15%) Absence of normal anatomical area of face. E.g. Loss of eye or part of nose. Visual or hearing loss will have to be separately evaluated.

Class 4-(15-35%) Impairment of whole person. Facial disfigurement is so severe that it precludes social acceptance.

This criterion appears logical, and it significantly simplifies an otherwise complex quantification of facial disfigurement. However, we would encourage its use with the other mentioned parameters. The multiple percentages can be resolved with the Kessler's formula.

In multiple disabilities and deformities or when there is a combination of the two, the Kessler's Formula can be used:

$$A + \frac{B\,(100-A)}{100}$$

Where A= the higher and B = lower value Another formula has also been used by Ramar as per the Government of India notification:

$$A + \frac{B\,(90-A)}{90},$$

again, A being the higher value and B being the lower value.

The formula can be used in a few mock situations.

1. X has an injury resulting in the fracture of the mandible and loss of four incisors. He also develops a paresis of the marginal mandibular nerve following surgery. His total percentile may be calculated thus: A = 15% and B = 5%.

$$15 + \frac{5\,(100-15)}{100} = 19.25,$$

whereas the sum of both would have been 20%.

2. Y has an injury resulting in the fracture of both condyles causing subsequent total bony ankylosis. He also has a large scar with keloid on his right cheek. His percentage is calculated thus:

$$50 + \frac{20\,(100-50)}{100} = 60$$

whereas the sum of two injuries would have 70.

Please note that the value adjusts itself as the percentile goes up.

5.3 Duties of Witness

After a warrant has been issued, it is possible to be held in contempt of court for not showing up in court without good cause.

Exaggeration or making false claims while on oath is not just immoral but also punishable by law (see Sections 181, 193, and 203).[1]

5.4 Conclusion

It is a huge undertaking to quantify various impairments and abnormalities. The only impairments that are the subject of this essay are those brought on by accidents. Congenital impairments/deformities, such as cleft lip and palate and craniofacial abnormalities, need a more thorough investigation. Similar to impairments and deformities brought on by aggressive tumors and malignancies of the head and neck, these issues might be global in nature. Particularly in the case of cancer, there might be a wide range of related issues, from morbidity at the donor site to problems with quality of life and mental distress.

Aesthetics and mastication are directly related to dental injuries, as well as the impairment or deformity that results from them. The anterior teeth were taken into account for beauty and the posterior teeth for masticatory function when determining percentiles. The rewards are arbitrary and based on the relative dysfunction brought on by the masticatory apparatus's lack of teeth. According to the recommendations of the American Association of Oral and Maxillofacial Surgery (AAOMS), percentages are given for the entire masticatory apparatus. It grants 24% for individuals who must only consume liquids (or 40%–60% if tube feeding is required) and 5–19% for those who must only consume semisolids (including those who can wear dentures).

We've gone ahead and given scores for certain teeth. However, if the entire masticatory system is to be assessed, one can assess each component independently, such as muscular strength, occlusal disharmony, TMJ mobility (craniomandibular articulation), and teeth loss. This Figure can then be calculated using Kessler's method.

$$A + \frac{B(100-A)}{100}$$

This formula, which takes into consideration specific limitations within the context of the masticatory apparatus, seems fair. Additionally, the AAOMS rules divide the percentiles into two groups.

1. The percentage of the norm.
2. The overall person's percentage of disability. The dichotomy fails to make sense and is probably going to lead to more misunderstanding. Finer features, including lateral excursion and other topics included in the AAOMS recommendations, were disregarded.

The AAOMS and the AMA recommendations have differing approaches to the concepts of deformity and disfigurement. Disfigurement is a complex topic that is made more difficult by problems like personality crises and the effects of societal acceptability. As previously mentioned, this criterion can be added to Kessler's formula to address the problem of various impairments and deformities. The issue of who can certify a disability is left until last. Regarding damage to the maxillofacial region, Indian sources are mute. However, a Board-certified Oral surgeon or Maxillofacial surgeon is required by law in several American states to give disability certification for the Maxillofacial area.

Contrary to popular belief, statutory entities are not required to create these requirements. Legal validity might come from common usage. Of course, it would be great if these recommendations could be examined, changed, and expanded to suit a wider range of impairments and deformities in order to benefit the surgeon, the patient, and the general public.

References:

1. N. S. Kedarnath et al. Maxillofacial Surgeon as Fact Witness for Medico-Legal Cases: Indian Scenario. J. Maxillofac. Oral Surg. (Oct–Dec 2015) 14(4):962–971

2. Jason Payne-James et al. Injury Assessment, Documentation, and Interpretation. Clinical Forensic Medicine: A Physician's Guide, 2nd Edition. Edited by: M. M. Stark © Humana Press Inc., Totowa, NJ.

Pathognomonic Signs of Death and Coma

6.1 Introduction

Verifying that death has actually happened is essential before issuing a death certificate. This can be difficult in the present era with sophisticated intensive care methods and the possibility of organ donation. There is currently no international agreement on what constitutes "death" and there is no legal definition of it in India. However, it is usually understood to signify *"the irreversible loss of capacity for consciousness combined with the irreversible loss of capacity to breathe"*.

Every nation provides instructions for diagnosis and death confirmation. [1] The Academy of Medical Royal Colleges' (2008) guideline primarily deals with death confirmation in hospitals and in circumstances in which determining the cause of death may be more challenging (those who are on ventilators, for example).

Death may be evident if there are evident pathognomonic markers (rigor mortis, hypostasis). If not, the evident signs of death should be noted by "the simultaneous and irreversible onset of apnea and unconsciousness in the absence of circulation".

The guidelines further suggest that:
Full and extensive attempts have been made, where appropriate, to reverse any underlying causes of the cardiorespiratory arrest, such as body temperature, endocrine, metabolic, and biochemical abnormalities that are more pertinent in a hospital setting.

One of the following conditions is met:
1. The person is exempt from trying cardiopulmonary resuscitation since they fulfil the requirements.
2. Cardiopulmonary resuscitation attempts have been unsuccessful.
3. Life-sustaining treatment has been discontinued because it has been determined that the patient will no longer benefit from it, that it is not in their best interest to carry on, and/or that it is in accordance with the patient's desires as expressed in a preliminary decision.

To ensure that an irreparable cardiorespiratory arrest has occurred, the person should watch the patient for at least five minutes. [2]

6.1.1 How to Verify Death (Figure 6.1)

It is important to perform a comprehensive physical examination to determine that a death has occurred. At first glance, there should be a severe pallor (especially on the face and lips), as well as relaxed facial muscles. If the eyelids haven't already been closed, this causes the lower jaw to drop and causes wide, glaring eyes.

- No perceptible pulses should be confirmed by further testing.
- Presence of asystole in the ECG
- Auscultation reveals no heartbeats
- No breathing effort noticed
- Auscultation reveals no breath sounds
- Pupils that are dilated and unresponsive to light

An exterior inspection of the body and the environment should be conducted, especially if the death was sudden, to check for any obvious circumstances that may have contributed to their demise (blood, vomit, wounds, weapons, alcohol, medications, written notes, etc.). For the certification of the exact cause of death, this is crucial. [3]

Another indication of death

- is lack of reaction to unpleasant stimuli.
- Reflexes in the cornea are absent.
- The cornea is cloudy.
- Evaluation of the trunk may reveal indications of hypostasis-related post-mortem staining.
- The possibility of rigor mortis (which starts around three hours following death) exists.
- Reduced temperature: this will depend on the surrounding temperature and might take up to eight hours.

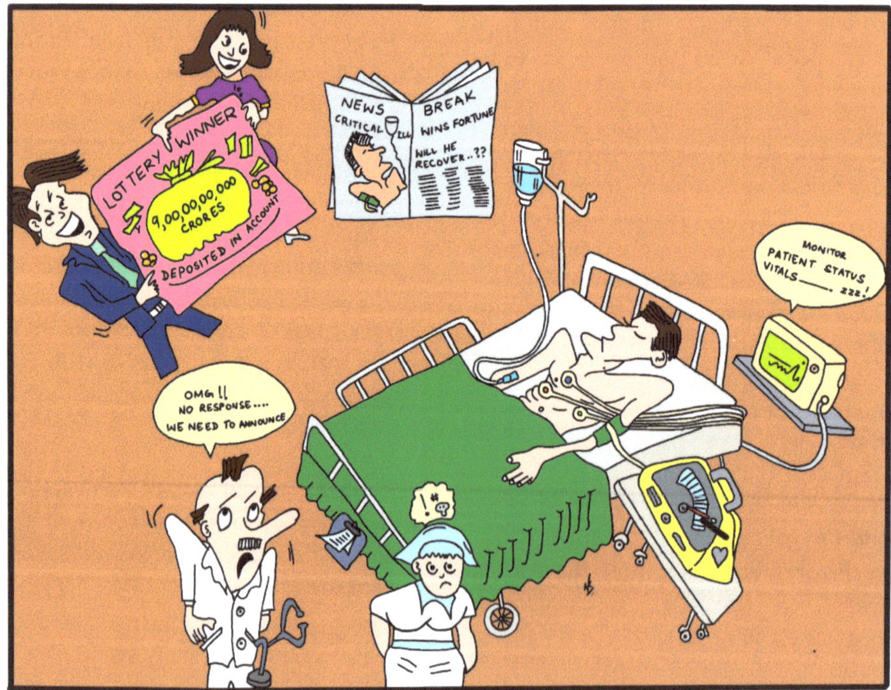

Figure 6.1: How to identify and confirm death

6.1.2 What to Do When the Precise Time of Death is Not Known

It may be challenging to pinpoint the exact moment of death, and an individual may still be resuscitated for some time after breathing and heartbeat have stopped.

If a patient is not carefully investigated, they may appear to be dead in the following situations:

- After drinking alcohol or using drugs,
- After extended immersion in cold water,
- While hypoglycemic or unconscious.

If they are given the proper care, they could fully recover. Resuscitation should be carried on in these situations as long as a typical body temperature is attained, regardless of whether the person being treated seems to be dead, because hypothermia shields against hypoxic damage to the nervous system, and children under the age of 5 tend to be more immune to hypoxic brain injury.

One can consider a circumstance where a child having paediatric craniofacial surgery has significant hypothermia following surgery, which results in cardiac arrest.

6.1.3 Practical Definition of Death in Primary Care

Death: Death is defined as the cessation of all vital functions of the body, including the heartbeat, brain activity (including the brain stem), and breathing.

Coma: Coma is a state of unconsciousness in which a person cannot be awakened; fails to respond normally to painful stimuli, light, or sound; lacks a normal wake-sleep cycle; and does not initiate voluntary actions. A person in a state of coma is described as being comatose.

GLASGOW COMA SCALE: It is a clinical scale used to reliably measure a person's level of consciousness in response to a defined stimulus. **(Table 1)**

Table 1: Glasgow coma scale

Behaviour	Response	Score
Eye opening response	Spontaneous	4
	To speech	3
	To pain	2
	No response	1
Verbal response	Oriented to time, place and person	5
	confused	4
	Inappropriate words	3
	Incomprehensible sounds	2
	No response	1
Motor response	Obeys commands	6
	Moves to localized pain	5
	Flexion withdrawal from pain	4
	Abnormal flexion (decorticate)	3
	Abnormal extension (decerebrate)	2
	No response	1
Total score	Best response	15
	Comatosed client	8 or less
	Totally unresponsive	3

The death may occur for different reasons. The type of death may vary depending on the cause of death. It is important to understand the definition of each form of death for final diagnosis before final declaration for the purpose of certification and understanding of the disease process.

Brain Death: The total and permanent loss of brain function, including the involuntary functions required to maintain life, is referred to as brain death.

Cardiac arrest: Cardiac arrest is the abrupt, unexpected loss of respiration, consciousness, and heart function. The most common cause of sudden cardiac arrest is an electrical disruption in the heart, which interferes with its ability to pump blood throughout the body.

Clinical death: Death determined by the medical observation of the loss of vital functions is referred to as clinical death. It is often recognized by the stoppage of breathing and pulse.

Vegetative state:

It is important to distinguish between issues with the diagnosis and treatment of vegetative states (VS) and issues with death. The VS, which has been described as a medical condition of being unaware of self and surroundings in which the individual breathes on their own, maintains stable blood pressure, and exhibits cycles of ocular opening and closing that may imitate sleep and wake, does not include brain-stem death.

For practical reasons in general practice, a patient who is unresponsive, has a body temperature over 35 °C, has not been using drugs or alcohol, and is not breathing on their own is often considered dead if:

- There aren't any unintentional motions.
- No respiratory effort is being made (look for at least a minute).
- There are no audible heartbeats or discernible pulses (look for at least a minute).
- Reflexes, including corneal ones, are absent.
- Pupils are dilated and fixed.

6.1.4 Pathognomonic Signs of Death

The precise mechanism of the reason for death and the physiology of the dying process must be fully understood whenever doctors are tasked with the responsibility of certifying a death. Although there are many conceptual sources available, the authors believed that understanding the real pathophysiology underlying each indication of death could be helpful for medical and dental professionals.

Although one may find all of these in other textbooks, the writers felt it was important to include this section in this textbook due to the new duty of death certification that a dental surgeon might be required to take on. It is even more crucial to have this conversation here due to the paucity of access to continuing medical education programs and the lack of this subject in dentistry's undergraduate and postgraduate curricula.

Given how simple it is to make a diagnosis using new technologies, it is very simple to disregard the art of clinical examination. Without invasive or expensive procedures, a rapid diagnosis can be made with a systematic cardiovascular examination. A thorough medical evaluation may produce a prompt and unanticipated diagnosis.

6.2 Clinical Signs of Death

6.2.1 Absence of Pulse (Pulselessness)

Radial pulse:
A pulse is the sensory arterial palpation of the heartbeat by fingertips. The brachial artery on the elbow, the carotid artery in the neck, the radial artery at the wrist, the popliteal artery in the knee, the femoral artery in the groin, the dorsalis pedis artery on the foot, and the posterior tibial artery around the ankle joint can all be used to palpate the pulse.

Pulse is the same as heart rate when expressed as the number of arterial pulses per minute. Auscultation, which is the process of actually hearing the heartbeat while utilizing a stethoscope, is another way to determine the heart rate.

Three fingers are typically used to measure the radial pulse: the finger most adjacent to the heart is used to obstruct the pulse pressure; the middle finger is used to cancel out the influence of the ulnar pulse because the two arteries are estimate of blood pressure; and the finger most distant from the heart (typically the ring connected by the palmar arches. **(Figure 6.2)**

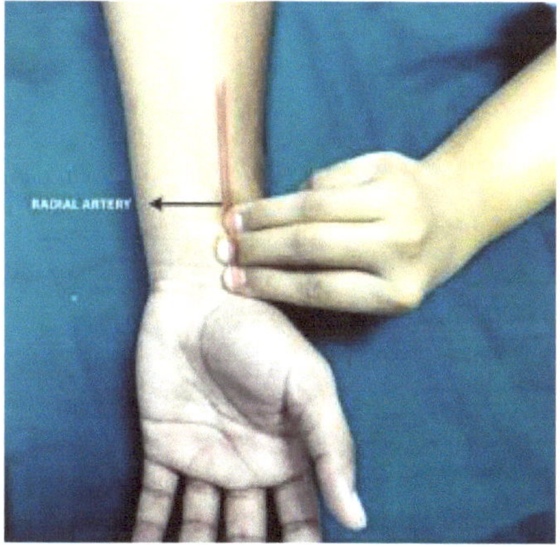

Figure 6.2: Method for checking the Radial pulse

Table 2: Normal pulse rates at rest, in beats per minute (BPM)

newborn (0–3 months old)	100-150
infants (3 – 6 months)	90–120
infants (6 – 12 months)	80-120
children (1 – 10 years)	70–130
children over 10 years & adults, including seniors	60–100
well-trained adult athletes	40–60

The lack of a pulse in the radial artery is one of the early signs of death. When simultaneous cardiac arrest results in death, you'll be able to feel or see a lack of pulse on the meter. When the heart stops pumping, there won't be a central pulse to feel, no heartbeat, and no breathing.

Carotid pulse:
In clinical settings, it is customary to start by checking the radial pulse. The routine assessment of the bigger brachial and carotid arteries to check for pulselessness, however, is highly advocated. The cause of this is that in individuals who are terminally sick or on the verge of death, a central pulse like the carotid pulse can be sensed from a greater artery than a collapsed peripheral radial pulse.

The examiner feels the movement of the artery wall caused by the pressure pulse as it passes by the point of palpation using the tactile or mechanoreceptors in their fingers. The fingers should be placed at the level of the cricoid cartilage, halfway across the larynx and the anterior portion of the sternocleidomastoid muscle **(Figure 6.3)**. The amount of pressure placed on the artery when palpating the pulse should be adjusted until the strongest pulsation is felt. Of course, there are special reasons to assess each pulse at each location as part of a thorough and organized cardiovascular examination. As always, there will be certain selectivity in clinical practice to speed up the final diagnosis and save time.

The arterial pulse displays the interplay of a driving force and a blood flow impedance. The heart's size and structure, heart rate, and the intrinsic contractility of the left ventricle all affect the driving power. The impedance is principally influenced by arterial compliance brought on by the distensibility of the vessel wall and peripheral resistance.

The aortic valve opens, releasing blood from the left ventricle to start the arterial pulse wave. As the blood reaches the aorta quicker than it is flowing to the peripheral vessels, the pressure in the pulse increases significantly. The left ventricle swiftly expels the majority of its stroke volume. The proximal aorta and other big central arteries, which are typically extremely distensible, temporarily hold a significant amount of this quickly expelled volume.

The absence of carotid pulse indicates that there is no left ventricular ejection, the driving force behind cardiac arrest, as there is no blood flow via the arteries.

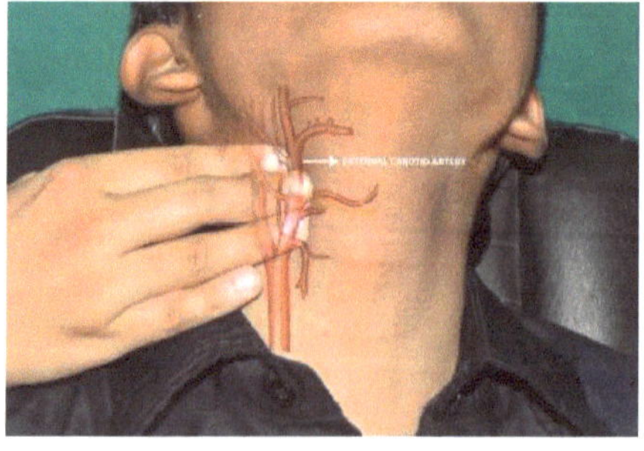

Figure 6.3: Method for checking the Carotid pulse

6.2.2 Absence of Heart Sounds

Due to the heart's lack of function, regular heart sounds are completely absent during auscultation. Nowadays, with easy access to cardiac catheterization and even echocardiography, it is possible to overlook the basic methods of auscultation of the heart.

The stethoscope's bell is better at picking up lower-frequency noises than its diaphragm is at picking up higher ones. The mitral valve and the diaphragm are often heard through the bell at all other locations.

6.2.3 No ECG Activity

A flat line on a monitor or ECG which denotes a cessation in electrical sequences and typically signifies a person's death, resembles a horizontal, straight line with an angle value of 180 degrees. **(Figure 6.4)**

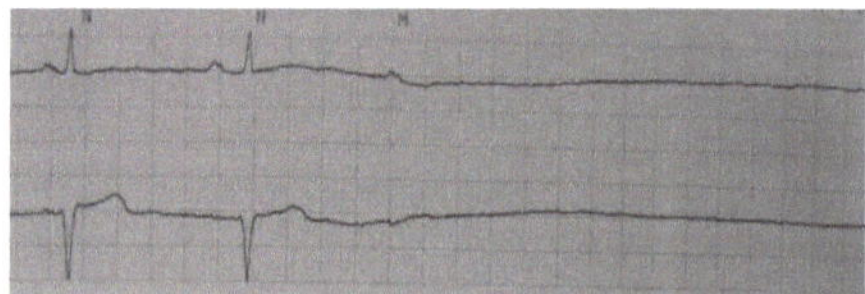

Figure 6.4: Couple of beats sinus rhythm followed by asystole in ECG

Electrical time sequence measurements that exhibit no activity produce flat lines instead of moving ones when they are shown. It nearly invariably refers to an ECG that is flat-lined, in which the heart does not electrically beat (asystole), or an electroencephalogram that is flat-lined, in which the brain does not electrically beat (brain death) **(Figure 6.5)**. These two particular incidents relate to different meanings of death in different ways. **(Figure 6.6)** depicts the normal pattern ECG.

Asystole is a condition of no cardiac electrical activity in medicine, which results in no myocardial contractions and no output from the heart or blood flow. One of the conditions that a doctor may utilize to confirm a patient's clinical or legal death is asystole.

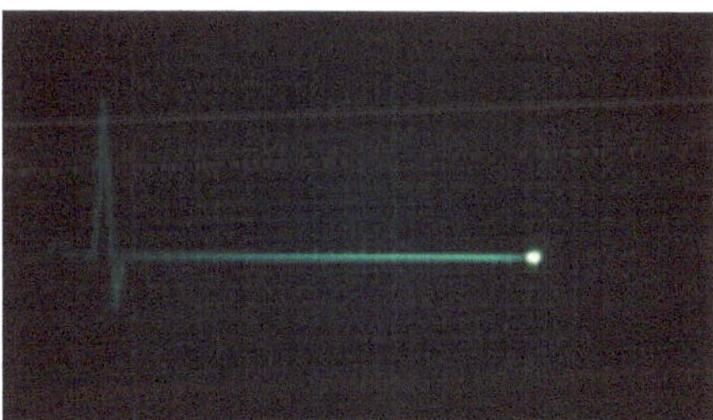

Figure 6.5: Flat line ECG pattern

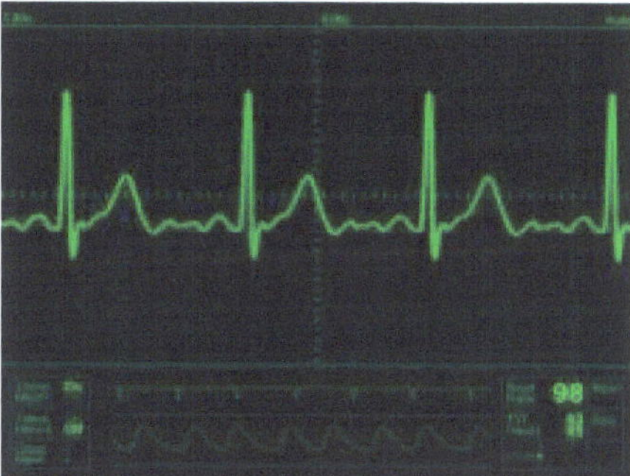

Figure 6.6: Normal ECG pattern

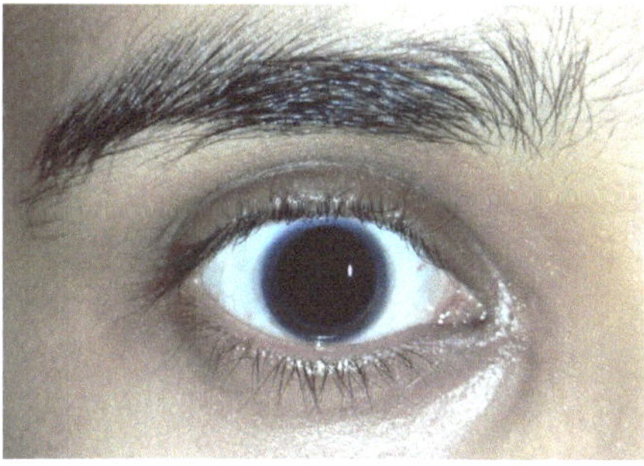

Figure 6.7: Illustrating fixed and dilated pupils

6.2.4 Pupils Unresponsive to Light

Fixed and dilated (**Figure 6.7**)

Pupillary Reflex Pathway (**Figure 6.8**)
When the parasympathetic nervous system is activated, the pupil closes, while sympathetic stimulation causes it to expand. As one of these systems is hindered, the reverse results. The size of the resting pupil reveals a balance between the two systems, based on the quantity of light or other factors like the supply of local or systemic medications.

The pupillary light reflex (PLR) is a reflex that controls the pupil's diameter in response to the intensity of light striking the retina of the pupil and the eye. The pupillary light reflex system is made up of an efferent limb (CN III) and an afferent limb (CN II). The ganglion cells of the retina can bilaterally access the pretectal nuclei.

To the Edinger-Westphal nucleus, which generates the preganglionic parasympathetic fibers, the pretectal nuclei project crossed and uncrossed fibers. These fibres connect to postganglionic parasympathetic neurons of the ciliary ganglion, which regulates the sphincter muscle of the iris, as they leave the midbrain with CN III.

The external or peripherally located pupillary fibres are sensitive to direct pressure and are often unaltered in an infarction of the nerve trunk (which can happen in diabetes), making it crucial to understand the microanatomy of these pathways. Eight to ten short ciliary nerves, which go around the eye to the constrictor muscle of the pupil, are produced by the ciliary ganglion.

The third cranial nerve, or the oculomotor, which supplies the constrictor muscles with nerve impulses, is lost upon death due to the lack of cranial nerve activity, which causes the pupils to dilate. The depletion of adenosine triphosphate (ATP) causes the pupils to stay fixed and dilated after death. The initial reaction after death is shown in the pupils. **Figure 6.8.1** depicts the difference between dilated and undilated pupil.

If severe, anoxia or ischaemia may result in fixed, dilated pupils. In experiments, acute anoxia causes pupillary constriction up to asystole or a cardiac output reduction of more than 70%, at which time the pupils open up and then close again 3 to 20 minutes following death.

Figure 6.8.2: Illustration of pupil dilation and contraction under dim and bright light

PUPILLARY LIGHT REFLEX

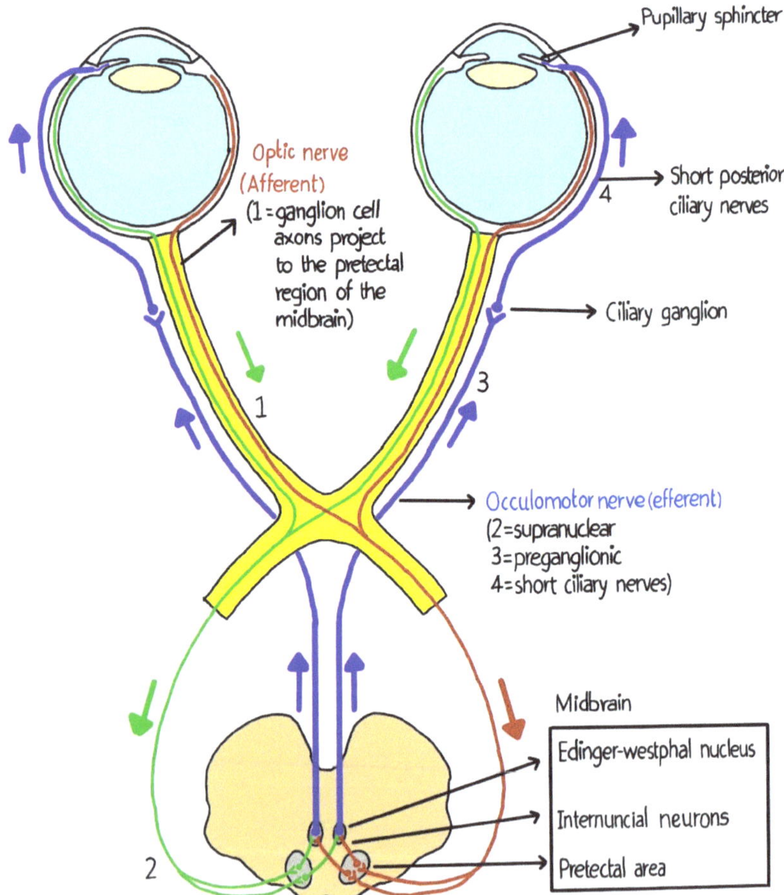

Figure 6.8: Pupillary Light Reflex

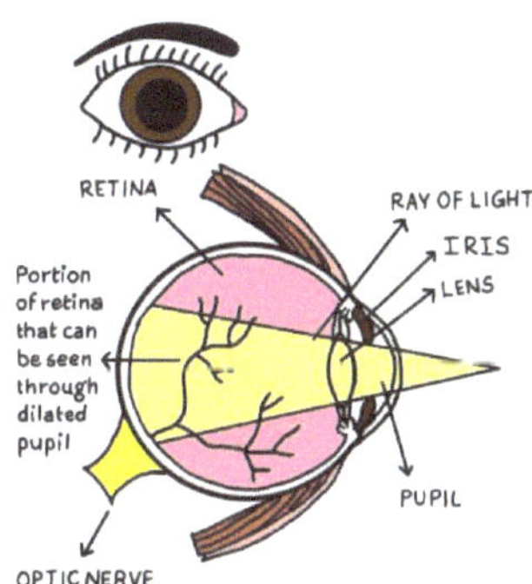

Figure 6.8.1: Depicting the difference between undilated and dilated pupil

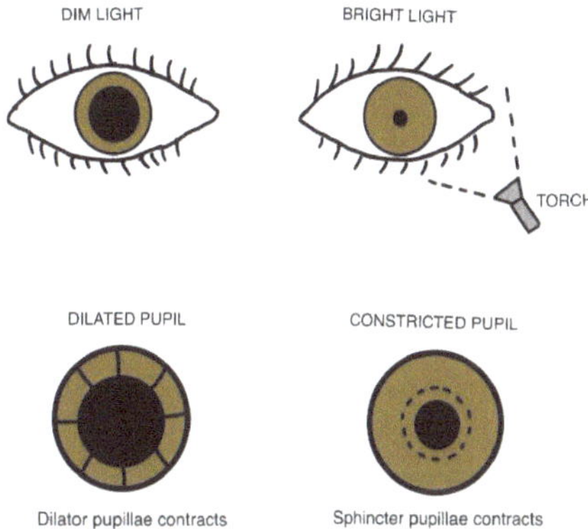

Figure 6.8.2: Illustration of pupil dilation and contraction under dim and bright light

6.2.5 Absence of Corneal Reflexes

The corneal reflex, which can be caused by any peripheral stimuli, is an automatic blinking of the eyelids that is triggered by activation of the cornea (such as by touching or by a foreign substance) or intense light. Both a direct and consensual response—the reaction of the opposing eye—should be elicited by stimulation. The reflex happens quickly, within 0.1 second.

This response, also known as the optical reflex, serves to shield the eyes from foreign objects and strong lights. Sounds that are louder than 40 to 60 dB can also cause the blink reflex to happen. The absence of a corneal reaction is proven by applying a cotton swab, tissue paper, or water squirts to the cornea. (**Figure 6.9**)

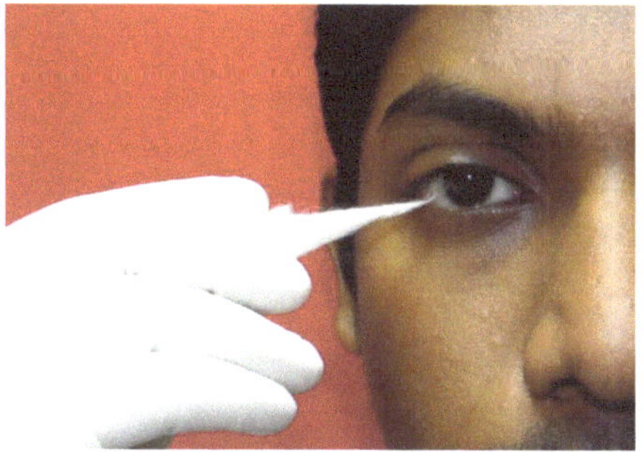

Figure 6.9: Test for corneal reflex by touching the cornea with a wisp of cotton and check for closure of eyelids

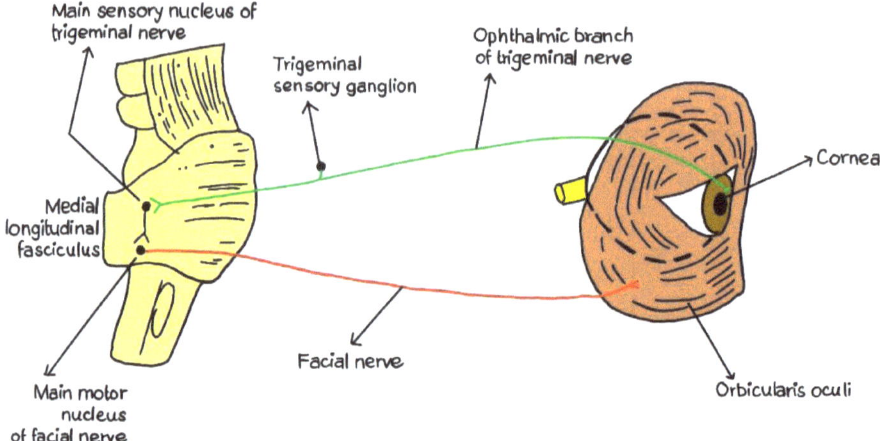

Figure 6.10: Corneal reflex pathway

Corneal reflex pathway:
The ophthalmic division of the trigeminal nerve carries afferent touch impulses from the cornea, or conjunctiva, to the sensory nucleus of the trigeminal nerve. Through the medial longitudinal fasciculus, internuncial neurons make contact with the motor nucleus of the facial nerve on both sides. The orbicularis oculi muscle, which causes the eyelid to close, is supplied by the facial nerve and its branches. **(Figure 6.10)**

This response is missing when the doctor uses a cotton swab to contact the cornea of a brain-dead patient to test it. The cranial nerves V and VII act as a conduit for this reaction.

6.2.6 Absence of Vestibulo-ocular Reflexes

The vestibulo-ocular reflex (VOR), occasionally referred to as but not quite synonymous with the oculocephalic reflex (which is also referred to as the "doll's head reflex" and is used, along with VOR, to evaluate the health of coma patients), is a reflex eye movement that triggers the vestibular system to cause eye movement.

By causing eye movements in the opposite direction of head movements, this reflex function preserves the picture in the centre of the visual field(s) during head movement, assisting in stabilizing images on the retinas (in yoked vision). For instance, the eyes shift to the left when the head goes to the right, and vice versa.

Once the head has rotated, the extraocular muscles on one side receive an inhibitory signal, and the muscles on the other side receive an excitatory signal. The eyes move to make up for the situation.

Oculo-vestibular reflex pathway
(Figure 6.11)
The vestibular system is the starting point of the route, where semicircular canals that are triggered by head rotation send impulses through Scarpa's ganglion and the vestibular nerve (cranial nerve VIII) to the vestibular nuclei in the brainstem. The contralateral cranial nerve VI nucleus (abducens nucleus) receives fibers from these nuclei. They connect with two more paths there. One of the paths uses the abducens nerve to transmit directly to the lateral rectus of the eye. A second nerve tract travels from the abducens nucleus

to the contralateral oculomotor nucleus through the medial longitudinal fasciculus. This nucleus is home to motor neurons that control eye muscle action, notably the medial rectus muscle of the eye. [4]

Patients who are brain-dead do not display a cold caloric reaction (oculo-vestibular reflex). When each tympanic membrane is irrigated with 50 cc of cold water successively while the patient's head is lifted at 30 degrees from a supine posture, there is no eye movement. **(Figure 6.12, Figure 6.13)**. The cranial nerves III, IV, VI, and VIII mediate this response.

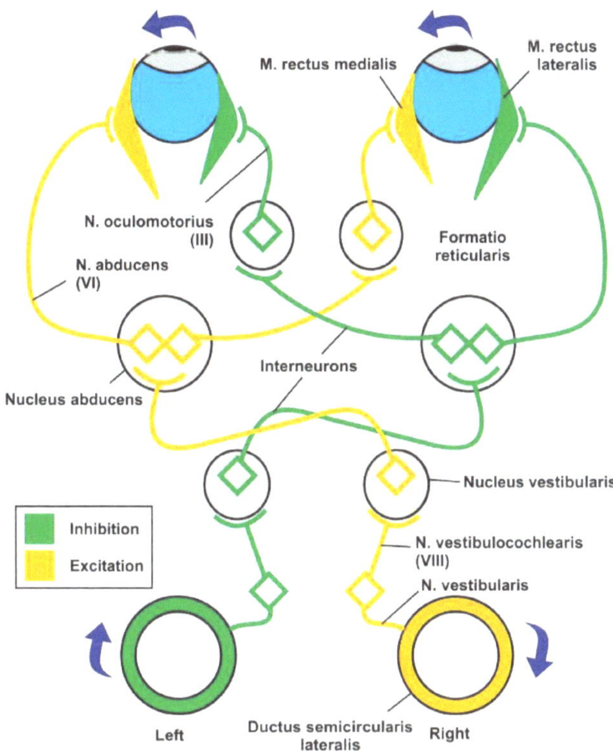

Figure 6.11: Oculo-vestibular reflex pathway

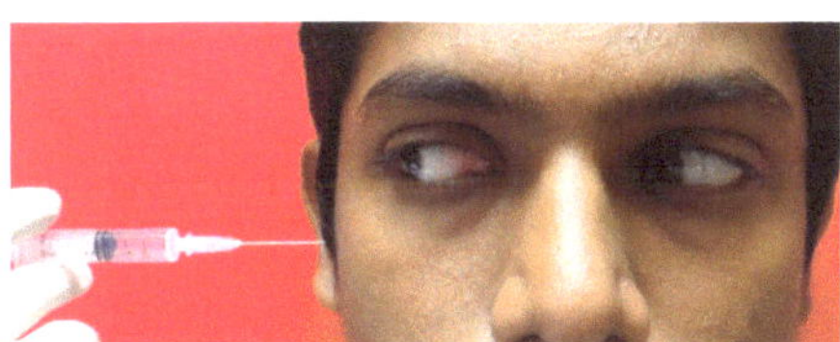

Figure 6.12: In a conscious patient, irrigation of the tympanic membrane with 50 cc of saline causes the eye to shift toward the side of the irrigation.

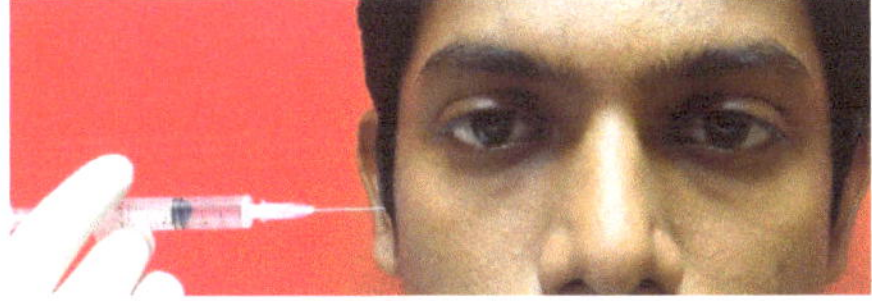

Figure 6.13: In brain dead individuals, irrigation of the tympanic membrane with 50 cc of saline causes no eye movement toward the irrigation side.

6.2.7 **Absence of the Gag or Cough Reflex**

The roof of the mouth, the back of the tongue, the region around the tonsils, and the back of the throat can all be touched to elicit the pharyngeal reaction, also known as the gag reflex or laryngeal spasm. Together with other aerodigestive reflexes like reflexive pharyngeal swallowing, it helps prevent choking by preventing objects from entering the throat, besides being part of regular swallowing.

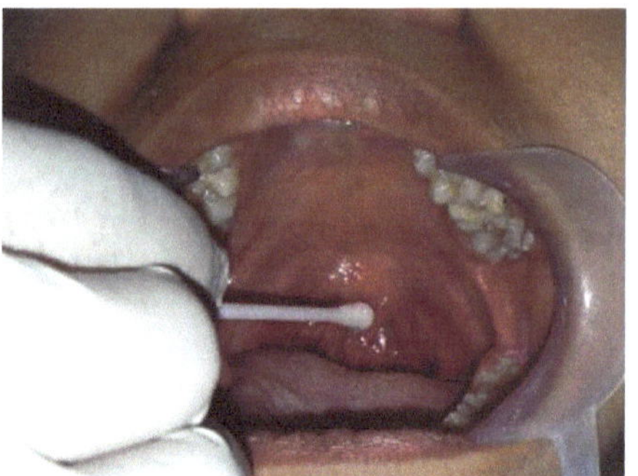

Figure 6.14: Inducing the gag response by stimulating the soft palate

Gag reflex pathway:
Many significant organs are innervated by the vagus nerve; however, the function of the throat, soft palate, and larynx must be tested in order to examine the nerve. By gently stroking the lateral wall of the pharynx with a spatula, the pharyngeal or gag reflex may be checked. The patient should start to vomit right away as a result of the pharynx muscles contracting. **(Figure 6.14)**

The glossopharyngeal nerve houses the pharyngeal reflex's afferent neuron, which travels to the stylopharyngeus muscle, and the vagus nerve, which travels to the pharyngeal constrictor muscles. [5]

When there is no retching or uvula movement after stroking the back of the throat with a tongue depressor or after repositioning the endotracheal tube in brain-dead patients, the gag reflex is absent. Cranial nerves IX and X control the gag reflex.

With deep tracheal irritation and suctioning, there is also no coughing. Cranial nerves IX and X control the cough reflex. No motor response is produced when the cranial nerve distribution is stimulated. **(Figure 6.15)**

6.2.8 **Trigemino-cardiac Reflex**

In both experimental animals and humans, electrical or mechanical stimulation of the trigeminal nerve causes a significant drop in heart rate, a noticeable drop in blood pressure, and apnea. The reflex reactions induced by stimulation of the trigeminal nerve are frequently referred to as the "trigeminocardiac reflex" and "trigeminal depressor responses" in the clinical literature.

The fast start of parasympathetic dysrhythmia, sympathetic hypotension, apnea, and/or stomach hypermotility upon activation of any of the sensory branches of the trigeminal nerve is known as the trigemino-cardiac reaction (TCR) **(Figure 6.16)**.

The reflex arc's afferent route is formed by the sensory nerve ends of the trigeminal nerve sending neuronal signals to the sensory nucleus of the trigeminal nerve through the Gasserian ganglion. To link with the efferent route in the motor nucleus of the vagus nerve, this afferent pathway travels further along the short internuncial nerve fibres in the reticular formation.

Also, during oro-facial and maxillofacial surgery, nasal fluid, mechanical stimulation of the eye and peri-ocular structures, and the oculo-cardiac reflex can all activate trigeminal afferent neurons. [6]

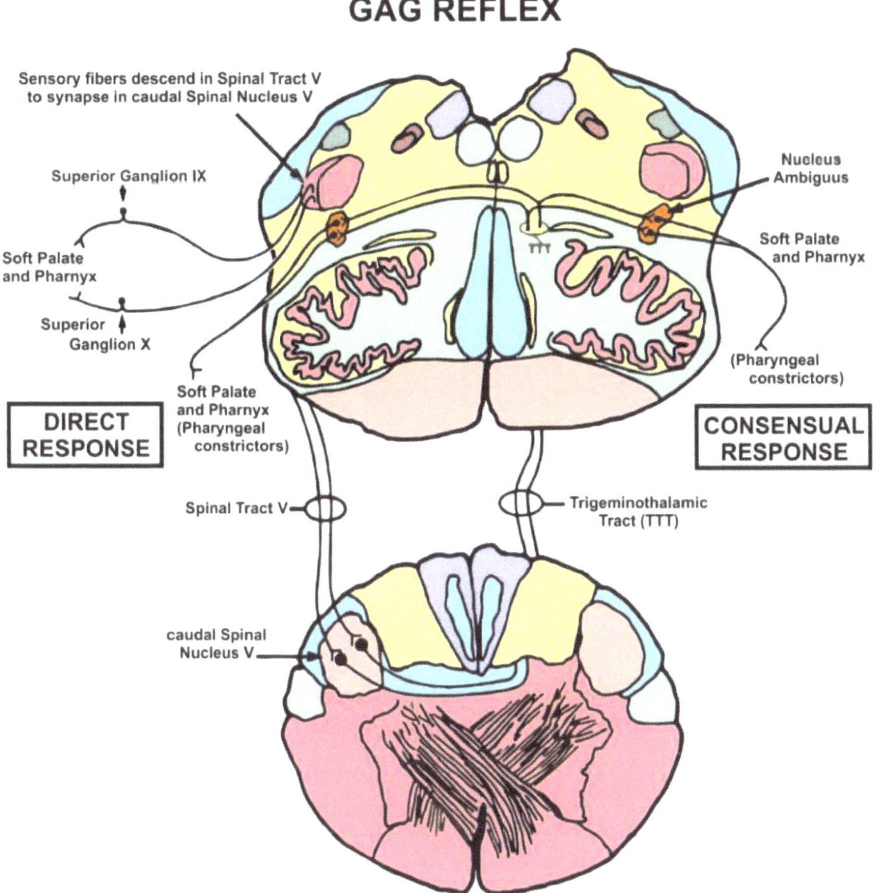

Touching of the soft palate and pharynx sends information to the ipsilateral caudal spinal nucleus V. Cells in spinal mucleus V project bilaterally to Nucleus Ambiguus resulting in elevation of the palate and gagging. The DIRECT response is on the same side as the stimulation, while the CONSENSUAL response is on the side opposite to the stimulus.

Figure 6.15: Gag reflex pathway

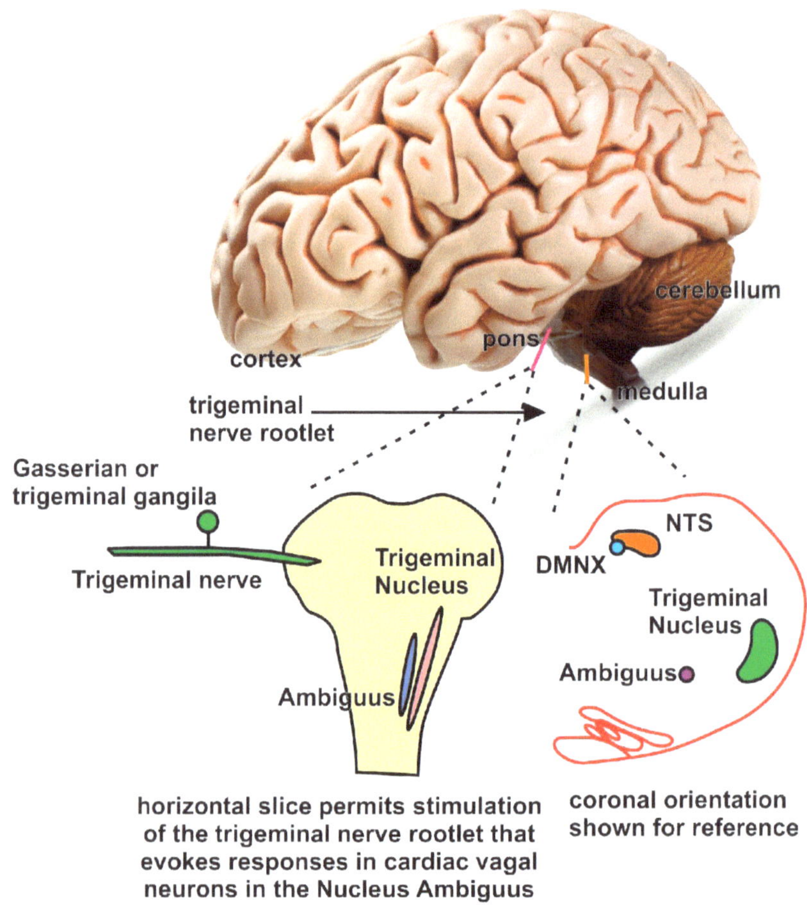

Figure 6.16: Trigemino-cardiac reflex

6.2.9 Oculo-cardiac Reflex

The oculo-cardiac reflex (**Figure 6.17**) is a phenomenon that develops as a result of activating extrinsic ocular muscles or moving a globe that is innervated by the trigeminal nerve's ophthalmic division.

The Aschner phenomenon, Aschner reflex, and Aschner-Dagnini reflex are other names for the oculocardiac reflex, which is a drop in heart rate brought on by pulling on the extraocular muscles or compressing the eyeball.

The reflex is mediated through nerve connections between the vagus nerve of the parasympathetic nervous system and the ophthalmic branch of the trigeminal cranial nerve via the ciliary ganglion.

These afferents connect to the brain stem's reticular formation's visceral motor nucleus, which is part of the vagus nerve. The vagus nerve transports the heart's efferent part from the cardiovascular region of the medulla, where increasing stimulation causes the sinoatrial node's output to decrease. [7]

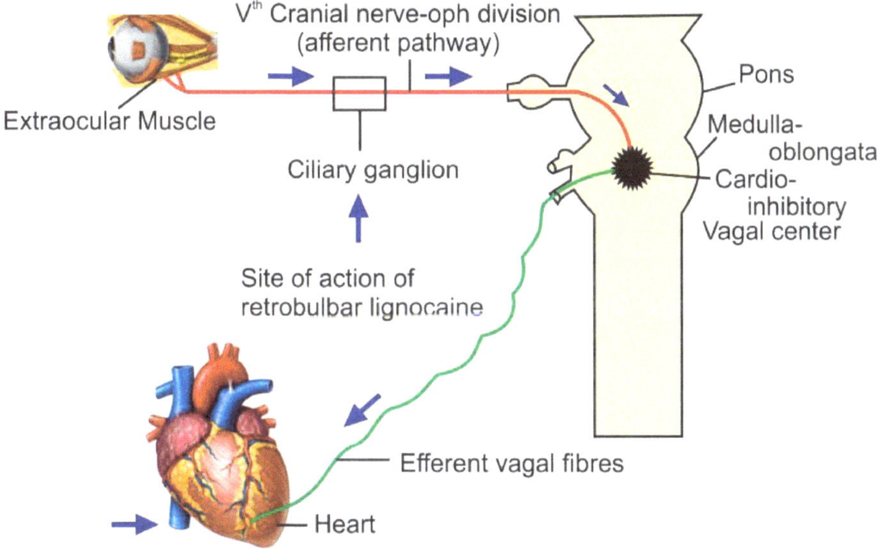

Figure 6.17: Occulocardiac reflex pathway

6.2.10 Apnea Test

The Apnea test (**Figure 6.18**) is a mandatory for determining brain death as it provides an essential sign of definitive loss of brainstem function. The respiratory response to an acidic stimulus is absent, and the breathing rate is decreased without causing hypoxia. The technique for assessing the brain-stem reflex for the respiratory reaction to hypercarbia (apnea test) ought to be the last one to be evaluated and should not be carried out if any of the earlier tests show that brain-stem reflexes are present. The procedure for performing the test and how frequently it should be done have both been the subject of debate in the past.

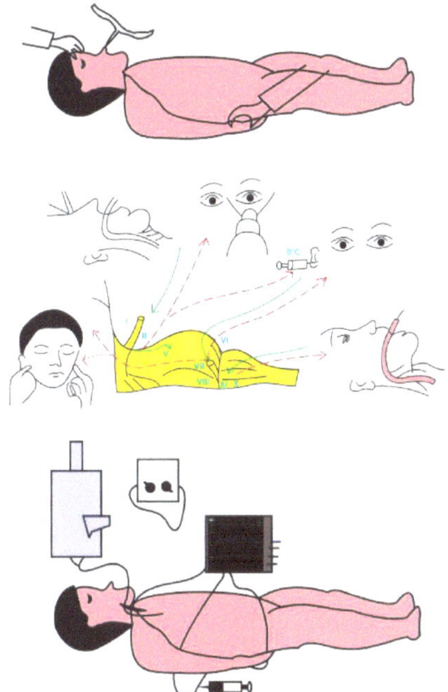

Figure 6.18: Apnea test

At least a consultant-level intensivist who is skilled in the administration and interpretation of brain-stem tests should make the diagnosis of death. One of the doctors must be a consultant at the very least. There must be no clinical conflicts of interest among those doing the testing, and neither physician may be a part of the transplant team. The designated doctors must work together to do the testing, and it must always be done twice. This is crucial for individuals with brain death whose families have consented to an organ donation.

There is a reason not to include the findings of neurophysiological or imaging studies as part of these criteria, given the reliability of the clinical criteria for determining the cause of death as a consequence of the termination of brain-stem reflexes during the previous thirty years. However, in situations where a thorough neurological examination is not possible (such as extensive facio-maxillary injuries, residual sedation, and some cases of paediatric hypoxic brain injury), in which a primary metabolic or pharmacological derangement can't be ruled out, or in situations where there is a high cervical cord injury, death cannot be determined solely by testing brain-stem reflexes. In these situations, a confirmatory test may eliminate any element of doubt and maybe minimize the length of observation needed before a formal assessment of the brain-stem reflexes.

The clinical algorithm for assessing collapsed patient has been described below in the form of a flow chart as a quick guide in emergency situations. **(Figure 6.19)**

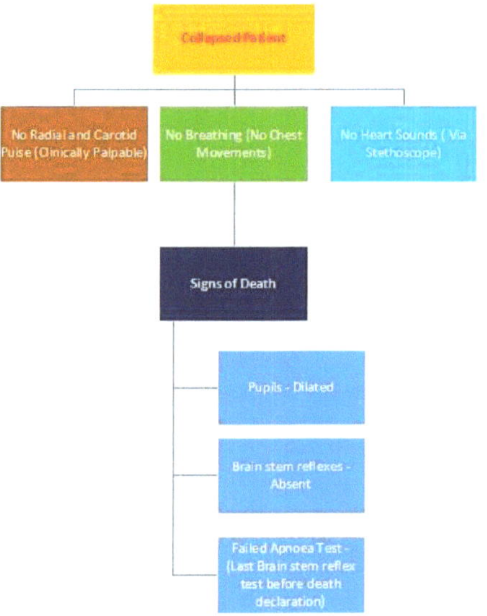

Figure 6.19: Algorithm for collapsed patient

Reference:

1. Gardiner D, Shemie S, Manara A, et al; International perspective on the diagnosis of death. Br J Anaesth. 2012 Jan108 Suppl 1:i14-28. doi: 10.1093/bja/aer397

2. Walker BR, Colledge NR. Davidson's principles and practice of medicine e-book. Elsevier Health Sciences; 2013 Dec 6.

3.   Scott JB et al. Apnea testing during brain death assessment: a review of clinical practice and published literature. Respir Care. 2013 Mar;58(3):532-8. doi: 10.4187/respcare.01962

4.   Fetter M. Vestibulo-ocular reflex. Dev Ophthalmol. 2007;40:35-51.

5.   Bensard D.D., Beauchamp K.M. (2012) Gag Reflex. In: Vincent JL., Hall J.B. (eds) Encyclopedia of Intensive Care Medicine. Springer, Berlin, Heidelberg

6.   Schaller B. Trigeminocardiac reflex. A clinical phenomenon or a new physiological entity? J Neurol. 2004 Jun;251(6):658-65.

7.   Yamashita M. Oculocardiac reflex and the anesthesiologist.Middle East J Anaesthesiol. 1986 Jun;8(5):399-415.

Responsibility of Dental Surgeons in the Event of Disability or Death

7.1 Introduction

This chapter is designed to acquaint dental surgeons and oral and maxillofacial surgeons with the vital death registration system in India and to provide instructions for completing and filing death certificates and death reports as required by the Registration of Births and Deaths (RBD) Act 1969. Emphasis is also given to the certification of medical information and issues relating to dental and maxillofacial events leading to morbidity or mortality.

A less significant number of medical deaths occur while patients are under the care of dental surgeons and oral and maxillofacial surgeons in India. The Dentist Act was silent on the issue of certifying death and/or cause of death. This is probably related to the issue not being relevant at the time of the Constitution of the Act (1948), when dentistry was a largely conservative and purely tooth-centric modality and death was not contemplated. Until recently, this issue was not addressed even in the amendments or regulations to the Dentist Act. With the advances and scope of dentistry being extended to include surgery and anaesthesia, the possibilities of acute events in the dental chair, operating rooms, and wards have increased exponentially. [1]

In the author's surgical career, it was very difficult to find an accurate explanation of procedures for carrying out the above-mentioned formalities. The dental curriculum, for obvious reasons, has not addressed these issues adequately in the past. This chapter attempts to correct this lacuna through a well-researched review of several sources, thereby providing sufficient information to the dental and maxillofacial surgeon in meeting the statutory requirements laid down by the Dental Council. The authors feel that this can only be achieved by exposing the dental surgeon to forensic medicine and by incorporating mandatory attendance at autopsies as part of their curriculum.

Although state laws minimally vary in specific requirements in India, almost 99% of the states follow the directions of the RBD Act guidelines for implementation and registration of death. [2]

Recent reports in the media about deaths in dental chairs, particularly with the use of dental anaesthesia, both local and sedation, have raised the issue of adequate knowledge of life support and causes of death.[3] It has become mandatory to impart better training in medical life support and reporting of adverse events.

At present, the spectrum of treatment offered by dental specialists and specialized maxillofacial surgeons have widened and include procedures such as complex implant procedures, oral oncology and reconstruction, complex mid-face operations for cleft and craniofacial syndromes, and complex trauma. The possibilities for dental-qualified persons encountering morbidity or mortality connected with these procedures have increased significantly. This is purely because, the more complex surgeries one undertakes, the chances of associated complications increase proportionately.

General dentists, including paediatric dentists, are increasingly using chairside conscious sedation and nitrous oxide anaesthesia for dental surgical work in the clinic environment. It is important that they are properly trained in the administration of anaesthetics and in managing emergencies arising from drugs and surgical procedures.[4] At this point, it is important to remember that in the unlikely event of a life-threatening emergency or death in an outpatient setting, the operator must know the protocols to be followed and the medico-legal implications of the procedures required.

The RBD Act lays down procedures for reporting death in a home and institutional setting. It lays down norms for reporting deaths in hospitals or while under the care of a health professional. India has a complex and pluralistic health care system that includes allopathy, Ayurveda, Unani, Siddha, etc., and each

of them is regulated by independent statutory bodies that train health professionals to deal with these situations as part of their curriculum.

Dental surgery falls under the broad practice of allopathy but has a separate regulatory body. Health professionals are therefore governed by different statutory bodies such as the Medical Council of India (now: National Medical Commission), AYUSH (Ayurveda, Yoga, Unnani, Siddha, etc.), and the Dental Council of India (now: National Dental Council). Each statutory body prescribes regulations for their respective practice and provides guidelines for practice, scope, and mandatory requirements, including eligibility, registration, and authority for various certifications.

In view of the fact that the recent regulations under the Dentists Act have redefined the scope of dental surgery and have outlined the duties of dental surgeons regarding disability and death, it has become important that all dental surgeons are kept well informed of the procedures to be followed in these situations.

This book's instructions are intended to help you correctly complete the **Medical Certificate of the Cause of Death (MCCD)**, report a death or disability, and act as a reference guide. Maxillofacial surgeons and dental professionals are the intended audience for this book. All dentists are advised to read this book before finishing their education, providing medical certificates of cause of death, or taking part in mortality and morbidity audits under the specified conditions. **Figure 7.1** illustrates medical and death audit.

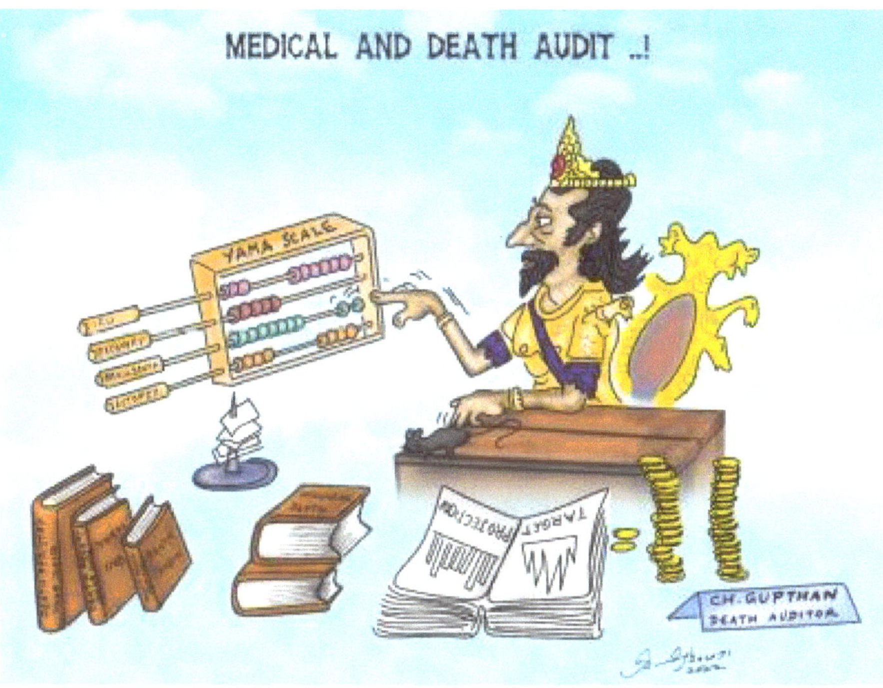

Figure 7.1: Medical and death audit

Death statistics are utilized for a variety of objectives by the federal, state (provincial), researchers, doctors, educational institutions, and many others. These consist of:

1. To evaluate the population's health state, the provision of healthcare, as well as shifts in state over time
2. To detect geographical variations in mortality rates, explore the causes of these variations, and research different types of fatalities
3. To keep an eye on changes in public health concerns such as newborn and mother mortality, infectious illnesses, accidents, suicides, and fatalities from carelessness, as well as accidents and infectious diseases.
4. To identify hazards connected to environmental, occupational, and general lifestyle aspects
5. To organize health facilities, services, and manpower;
6. To prioritize and allocate resources for health research and treatment;
7. To develop preventative and screening programs; and to evaluate the effectiveness of these programs.
8. To create health promotion initiatives and assess their outcomes.

7.2 Responsibilities of Dental Surgeons for Acute Morbidity or Mortality in the Dental Clinic and Hospitals

A healthy death is not a single event; rather, it is a sequence of occasions, connections, and long-term planning. There is no universal definition of what makes for a decent death; instead, excellent care has to be negotiated to take into account the unique values and preferences of each patient.

Death and morbidity in a dental clinic due to dental treatment are rare, as dental clinics do not routinely perform complex invasive procedures. However, we do hear of deaths due to morbidities such as cerebrovascular accidents (CVA), myocardial infarctions, hypotension due to adrenal crisis, etc. In general, cerebrovascular dental patients today are much older, and many of them have co-morbid conditions like cardiac, respiratory, and neurological diseases. Many of them are receiving drugs that might have consequences for procedures. Conscious sedation and drugs used for medication can also sometimes be lethal.

The dentist should be geared up to deal with morbid situations. The clinic must be adequately prepared for such eventualities with appropriate monitors, diagnostic equipment, drugs, and resuscitative equipment for patients who may develop medical emergencies. Most importantly, all clinics must have protocols and algorithms to deal with contingencies, including death. A comprehensive list of equipment and drugs needed in dental outpatient clinics is discussed in Chapter 2. This chapter briefly outlines procedures for reporting and referring patients with acute medical conditions or death in the dental office.

7.2.1 Acute Medical Conditions

It is the responsibility of every healthcare provider to attend to a sick patient and provide emergency life-saving measures like cardiopulmonary resuscitation (CPR), etc., before transporting the patient. In the event of a serious medical event, the dental surgeon must immediately call for emergency transfer of the patient to a full-fledged intensive care facility in a hospital. In the meantime, the dentist must institute all emergency procedures outlined for the condition. He should not leave the side of the patient until they are transferred to a hospital facility or competent care.

A careful diagnosis must be made with the available aids, and the patient must be stabilized as per protocol. An assistant should record all vital signs and make an entry of all the events and interventions done by the dentist. The shifting and positioning of patients should be as per protocol. The dentist should, to the best of their ability, provide a complete and detailed report of the events, including vital signs, provisional diagnosis, first aid, and drugs used. This will be helpful for the intensivist or emergency physician to further stabilize the patient.

The details of appropriate resuscitation and drugs for various conditions are mentioned in Chapter 3 - *Guidelines for Training of Dental Specialists in Basic Resuscitation Courses and for Emergency Management.*

7.2.2 Death in the Dental Clinic or Practice

Death in a dental clinic can occur for several reasons. It may be a death due to a pre-existing morbid condition like ischemic heart disease or an anaphylaxis/ toxicity anaphylaxis, cerebrovascular accident. On the other hand, it may be due to the exacerbation of an existing condition due to stress or pain. Several drugs used in dentistry can potentially cause death, e.g., anaphylaxis or toxicity from drug overdose. Obstruction of the airway due to infection or a foreign body and aspiration into the respiratory tract are also possible. Other rare possibilities include exsanguination from high-flow central hemangiomas or in persons with severe bleeding disorders. However, the most common cause of death in a dental chair is complications resulting from conscious sedation or outpatient short GA in western countries.[5] However, in India general anaesthesia in dental chair is not permitted and practised.

If the dental surgeon is certain of the occurrence of death after due recorded monitoring of vital signs and failure to respond to standard resuscitation protocols, he should proceed with[6]:

1. Information to the police. It must be remembered that all deaths within 7 days of treatment are deemed to be unnatural and therefore have medico-legal implications. The sudden death of an ambulatory patient in a dental clinic must therefore be construed as an unnatural death. Any such death will be brought to the notice of the police, either as a complaint or it may be taken up suo motto by the nearest police station. However, the best way is for the dentist to directly inform the police. This will prevent social discord and emotional issues. A declaration of death should be made after confirmation. If in doubt, the patient may be shifted to a hospital facility.

2. Once a complaint is filed or the police take suo moto cognizance, an FIR (first information report) will be registered. If there is a complaint of negligence, then the FIR will be filed under Section 304A (a rash and negligent act resulting in death).

3. Section 304A is cognizable, bailable, and non-compoundable. However, a Supreme Court ruling in *Jacob Mathew vs. Union of India 2005* prohibits any arbitrary arrest of a doctor without a credible medical opinion from a board set up for the purpose. The body of the deceased should thereafter be handed over to the police and sent for autopsy after declaring death and entering only the known reason for the cause of death. If the reason is unknown, the cause of death can be left blank.

4. An autopsy or post-mortem is performed in designated government or other hospitals, and the autopsy report will ascertain the cause of death.

5. Duly constituted medical boards can decide on issues of negligence if a 304A case is registered.

6. If there are no complaints by the next of kin (NOK) or family/relatives, the Medical Cause of Death Certificate is completed and submitted to the appropriate registration office for birth and death, and a tear-away slip or copy of the MCCD certificate is given to the NOK or family with the signature of the last health care provider.

7.2.3 Death in Hospitals

This is a less frequent incident and is usually encountered by dental surgeons specializing in oral and maxillofacial surgery who perform major surgical procedures under GA or attend to patients who have serious co-morbidity like head injuries, systemic diseases, or severe life-threatening infections that contribute to morbidity or mortality.[7,8]

Most hospitals have clear protocols for declaring death and issuing cause-of-death certificates. Standard forms are available for recording death, handing over of the body to relatives or police (as the case may be), receipts from the police, and morbidity and mortality log records.

If the Maxillofacial surgeon is the treating doctor and the patient has been admitted under him/her, then it is their responsibility to surgically intervene, institute emergency resuscitation, and make appropriate references to declare death in the unfortunate event that everything fails.[9] As per the RBD, the attending doctor (or any competent person designated by the hospital) must declare death and fill out the Medical Certificate of Cause of Death (MCCD). The details are referred to in Chapter 10- *Autopsy and Forensic Medicine*. In cases where the cause is not certain, it may be left blank to be ascertained by other means, including a postmortem examination or autopsy. Unnatural deaths, deaths due to accidents, peri-operative deaths, or deaths occurring unexpectedly within 7 days of being under the care of a doctor must be declared and certified by the attending doctor before handing the body for postmortem or forensic examination to ascertain the exact cause. The details of forms and records for doing so are discussed in the further chapters.

References:

1. L.M.Worthington et al. Death in dental chair: an avoidable catastrophe?. British journal of anaesthesia. Vol 80, No.2. Feb 1998

2. Jevon P (2013). Basic guide to Medical emergencies in the Dental Practice. 2nd Ed, Wiley Blackwell, Oxford.

3. Somnath Das et al. Medical Audit and Death Audit. J Indian Acad Forensic Med, 32(4)

4. Joginder Pal Attri et al. Conscious Sedation: Emerging Trends in Pediatric Dentistry. Anesth Essays Res. 2017 Apr-Jun; 11(2): 277–281.

5. Helen H. Lee et al. Trends in Death Associated with Pediatric Dental Sedation and General Anesthesia Paediatr Anaesth. 2013 August; 23(8): 741–746. doi:10.1111/pan.12210.

6. Evans N, Walsh H. The organization death and dying in todays society: Nursing standard. 2002; Vol.16: 33-38

7. Coplans MP, Curson I. Deaths associated with dentistry. *British Dental Journal* 1982; 153: 357–62.

8. https://indiacode.nic.in/

9. Jacob Mathew v. State of Punjab, the judgment stipulates the guidelines to be followed before launching a prosecution against a doctor for negligence. J Neurosci Rural Pract. 2013 Jan-Mar; 4(1): 99–100.

Procedures for Reporting Death by Dental Surgeons

8.1   Introduction

8.1.1   Death Certification

The RBD Act established a hierarchical structure for the nation's registration apparatus, with the Registrar General of India at the Centre serving as its head. The principal executive authority in the state responsible for carrying out the Act's requirements is the principal registrar of births and deaths. For documenting births and deaths that take place in the area assigned to them within a district, there are district registrars, registrars, and sub-registrars. To carry out the parts of the Registration of Births and Deaths Act, the States have created rules in line with the Model Rules with the Central Government's permission. [1,2]

The purpose of this chapter is to familiarize dental, oral and maxillofacial surgeons with India's mandatory death registration system and to offer guidelines for filling out and submitting MCCD and death reports. When they fall under the purview of the medical-legal officer, emphasis is also placed on the authentication of medical data and matters connected to such dental and maxillofacial occurrences.

The authors attempt to give the best information to those doctors or dental specialists coming under the ambit of dental specialty and provide them with enough information to complete the process of declaration and certification of cause of death using the correct procedure so that the registration authorities may issue a death certificate. Since the dental curriculum does not explicitly provide information for the formalities involved in a situation of death, this book will endeavour to concisely address the issue in accordance with the requirements of the regulations passed by the Code of Ethics pertaining to the issuance of certificates for disability and death while under the care of a dental specialist or oral and maxillofacial surgeon. The Dental Council is now obliged to provide training in these areas of forensic medicine and toxicology.

Recent reports in the media about outpatient mortality, specifically in children, have sparked a lot of confusion among dental professionals about how to proceed when such an event happens in a dental chair. Knowledge of death and its causes, identification, and good certification are therefore mandatory for accurate registration of events.

Dental anaesthesia, including those for paediatric dental management, has increased the risk of morbid events. Dental clinics and dental surgeons therefore need to be trained to recognize emergency situations and resuscitate patients who are in danger.

At this point, it is important to remember that most deaths in dental chairs occur intraoperatively or perioperatively.

Purpose and importance of death certification:
Central and state governments, researchers, clinicians, educational institutions, and others use death statistical data for many purposes.

These include:

1. To discover geographical variations in mortality rates, explore the origins of these variations, and research different reasons for death
2. To evaluate the population's health state, the provision of healthcare, and changes in that status over time.
3. To understand various reasons why mortality occurred in the dental field and how to prevent it in the future
4. To keep an eye on changes in public health concerns such as baby and maternal mortality, infectious illnesses, accidents, suicides, and fatalities from carelessness.
5. To identify hazards related to general lifestyle, environmental, and occupational variables
6. To prioritize and allocate resources for health research and healthcare;
7. To design health facilities, services, and human resources;
8. To organize preventative and screening programs and evaluate the outcomes of these programs.
9. To create health promotion initiatives and assess the outcomes.
10. Request for a grant from the government for specific aspects of the death cause study

8.1.2 Unnatural Deaths

If there is evidence to suspect that a person died from a cause other than sickness or as a result of someone else's carelessness, malpractice, or wrongdoing, examine the likelihood of a death that was unnatural. Such conditions could require an inquiry.

- ***Accidental Mortality***: A serious maxillofacial injury, for instance, that occurs before a fatal medical condition, such as aspiration pneumonia, is regarded as non-natural. There must be a forensic and legal examination of the body.
- ***Foreign body aspiration***: If a patient who had treatment from a dentist dies in the clinic or at home due to an aspiration of a foreign body, like small removable acrylic dentures dislodged into the larynx or vocal cord area, leading to asphyxiation, there is a potential for legal consequences and must therefore be subject to a forensic investigation.
- ***Sudden and unexpected death***: The sudden death of a patient due to unknown causes or underlying co-morbidities may need forensic investigation if there is a doubt. However, if the patient was moribund or known to be very sick, it may not need a forensic investigation as long as the patient's relatives and next of kin are satisfied that it was natural.
- It is advisable to conduct a forensic inquiry if family members express uncertainty or if there have been disputes about treatment choices.

Birth and death are inexorably linked and follow each other. Life is the intervening period.

The death certificate is a permanent record that life has ceased. The record's details are regarded as sufficient proof of the fact of death, and the treating doctor or forensic pathologist must provide a reasonable cause for such an event, which in turn can be used for administrative or legal purposes. [3]

8.2.1 Dental Surgeons as Certifiers

Whenever a dental surgeon encounters a death in a dental chair, in a private hospital, or while employed in a government hospital, the principal responsibility in death registration is to complete the Medical Cause of Death Certificate (MCCD), whenever required.

By giving closure with a thorough and full certification that will enable the family and authorities to conclude the person's affairs, the dental surgeon fulfils the job of the certifier and provides the final act of care to a patient.

When he is the final caregiver, the dentist's responsibility will be:

1. To be knowledgeable of federal, state, and local laws governing the certification of medical causes of death

2. To the greatest extent of their knowledge, complete the pertinent sections of the MCCD.

3. Promptly hand over the certified document that has been signed and authenticated to the relative so that they can apply for a death certificate from the neighbourhood authorities and provide the relevant information for the ultimate disposition of the remains.

4. Support the state or local registrar by swiftly responding to questions.

5. When autopsy results or additional investigation show the cause of death to be different from what was initially reported, provide a supplementary report of the cause of death to the state vital statistics office.

When a death occurs in a hospital or other institution, several states permit that facility to begin the process of preparing the death certificate. In these situations, the attending oral and maxillofacial surgeons or dental surgeons can often finish and sign the cause-of-death part of the certificate at the hospital or other institution.

Another competent person on duty at the hospital or other institution may declare the deceased as legally dead and may permit release of the body to the next of kin when the participating dental surgeons (dental surgeons in charge of the patient's care for the condition that resulted in death) are not available to certify the cause of death at the time of death. The attending dental surgeon will verify the cause of death in such situations later.

Dental surgeons are required to certify the cause of death if they are the patient's final healthcare provider. Only when state law allows for another appropriate entity (competent person) to do the task of declaring death, if the attending oral surgeon is unable to declare the cause of death at the moment of death. [4]

If not done correctly, there can be information gaps, especially when it comes to the cause of death. Determining the cause of death and the manner of death is crucial because doctors, attorneys, and members of the general public sometimes have trouble distinguishing between cause of death, mechanism of death, and manner of death.

8.2.2 **Cause of Death**

Any illness or injury that causes a physiological imbalance in the body and ultimately leads to death is referred to as a fatal physiological imbalance. For instance, a neck adenocarcinoma or a headshot wound.

Mechanism of death:
The physiological disturbance brought on by the cause of death, which causes death, is the mechanism of death.

For instance, a hemorrhage, septicemia, lung metastases, etc.

Cause of death:
The reason for death is explained by the method of death. The most common causes of death include natural homicide, suicide, accidents, and undetected or undeclared causes. Therefore, just as a cause of death might have several causes and numerous mechanisms.

In order to confirm the details listed on a death certificate or to explain what was meant, the dental surgeons will be called. From a clinical perspective, the first cause-of-death declaration might not be incorrect, but it could not contain enough details.

The rate with which a dental surgeon has to devote extra time to responding to follow-up queries concerning a patient's cause of death should be reduced by adhering to the instructions in this manual.

The vital statistics system includes mortality statistics as a crucial component. For administrators and health professionals to evaluate the efficacy of the public health services they deliver, accurate medical certification and records are crucial (**Figure 8.1**). They offer input for future health department policy and execution, and they are also crucial for medical research projects.

Analysis of the cause of death in vital statistics data is a critical step in developing national and state health policies and programs, and it has a significant impact on the quality of public health services. An accurate medical certification of the cause of death is also necessary for practical matters like hospital reimbursement, life insurance claims, obtaining a probate or succession certificate, settling property claims, releasing gratuity and provident fund claims, removing the deceased's name from the ration card and voter list, and ratifying pension plans.

8.2.3 **Legal Provisions**

The Registration of Births and Deaths Act (RBD) of 1969 was enacted by the Indian government and requires confirmation from a doctor or other healthcare professional who treated the dead during his or her final illness. According to the law, the reason for a death should be documented concurrently with its occurrence since both are crucial.

The top authority in India, the Registrar General, is responsible for compiling data on births and deaths from cantonment boards of military cantonments, municipal corporations and municipalities of towns, and registrars and sub-registrars of births and deaths at the district level.

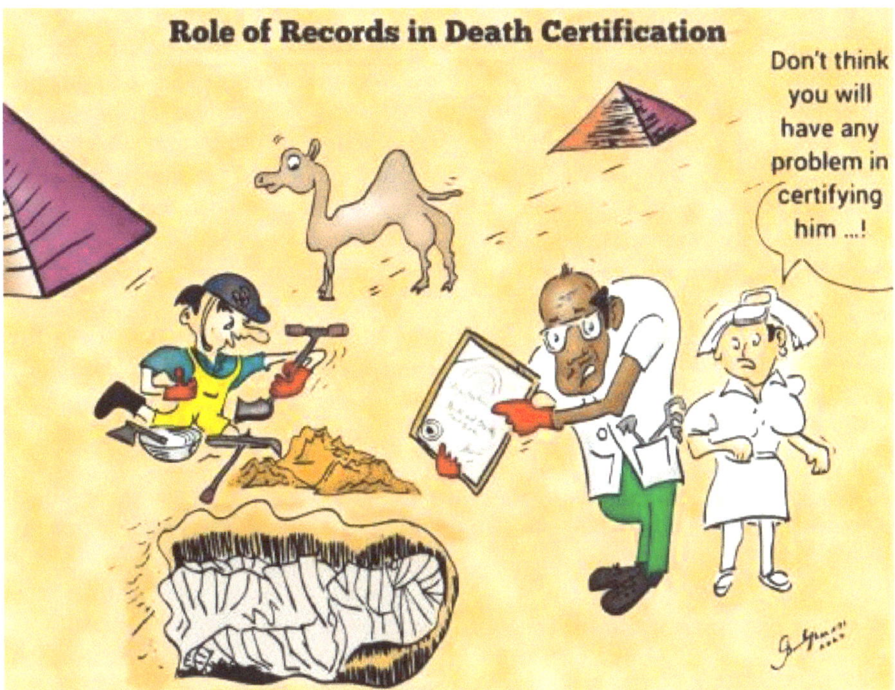

Figure 8.1: Role of records in death certification

A pragmatic change in records was made for data collection, review, and statistical analysis for the Registrar General of India after various commissions and committees examined the Indian vital statistics system following independence.

In India, medical certification of cause of death (MCCD) is carried out in accordance with the government medical certification plan, a program put in place by the relevant state governments that also involves training for medical professionals. Although MCCD is sometimes referred to as a "death certificate," the two are distinct. Both are of crucial legal and medical relevance. The effects of incorrect filling brought on by ignorance or disregard are extensive.

8.2.4 Importance of Death Certification

MCCD is crucial for claiming family allowance, hospital reimbursement, life insurance, obtaining a probate or succession certificate, settling inheritance or property claims, making gratuity and provident fund claims, and removing the deceased person's name from ration cards, employer registers, etc. It also serves as a legal and protective measure.

Administrative purposes: Documenting the cause of death can be used to identify contagious and epidemic illnesses that need to be controlled. It could also show whether any adjustments need to be made in the way public health services are provided. It aids in the avoidance of accidents, the execution of eradication plans, and the upkeep of illness case records, social security records, and tax registers.

Utilization in statistics: Understanding the patterns in mortality by age, sex, and cause is essential for developing and assessing health care development strategies. As a result, the registration records are most valuable as legal documentation and secondarily as a source of vital data.

8.2.5 Legal Provisions

Sections 10(2) and 10(3) of the Registration of Births and Deaths Act of 1969 provide statutory support for medical certification of cause of death under the civil registration system. [5-7]

A certificate relating to the cause of death must be acquired by the registrar from such a person and in such a form as may be required, according to Section 10(2) in any region, the state government having respect for the facilities therein in this regard.

In the event that a person who was receiving medical care during his or her last illness passes away in a state where the government has mandated that a certificate as to the cause be obtained, Section 10(3) states that the state government shall immediately issue, free of charge, to the person required by this act to provide information regarding the death, a certificate in the prescribed form stating, to the best of his or her knowledge.

The registrar, after making the necessary entries in the register of births and deaths, forwards the certificates to the chief registrar or officer deputed by him by the *10th of every month,* subsequent to the month when the certificate was issued.

Any individual may acquire an extract pertaining to death by paying the required fees to the government, according to Section 17(1)(b) of the Registration of Birth and Death Act. However, unless it is in the best interests of the general public, the reason for death will not be made public.

Even though this is typically done through a relative of the deceased, who only receives permission from the municipality to dispose of the dead body after demonstrating the death certificate for registration in accordance with the RBD act, it is the responsibility of the signing medical or dental practitioner to send the death certificate to the registering authority.

Any medical professional who neglects or refuses to issue a certificate under Section 10(3) and any person who neglects or refuses to deliver such a certificate are both subject to fines under Section 23(3) of the RBD Act, which may be determined by state government regulations. [5]

8.2.6 Registration of Death

The identification of the dead, the date and time of death, and the reason for death must be given to the registration authorities in order to record a death. The registration of Births and Deaths (amendment) Act, 2023 mandates all the states to digitally register births and deaths on the Centre's Civil Registration System (CRS) portal and share data with the RGI which functions under the Union Home Ministry from October 1st 2023. Death cannot be reported if any of this information is missing. For instance, in the United Kingdom, a physician can't verify death and fill out the reason for death until he is dealing with the patient in the latter stages of death, or the dead should have been in his care and treatment for at least 15 days prior to the patient's death.

Due to a number of factors, the cause of certain fatalities may not always be known. With the family's permission, a clinical postmortem is performed in certain cases to determine the cause of death.

A postmortem is performed during the course of the inquest in complicated medicolegal matters in order to determine the deceased's identification, cause of death, and time of death. The cause of death may only be determined by a postmortem performed by a qualified and authorized medical official; however, they may also take autopsy tissues to aid in the inquiry if the medical case warrants it. [5] **(Figure 8.2)**

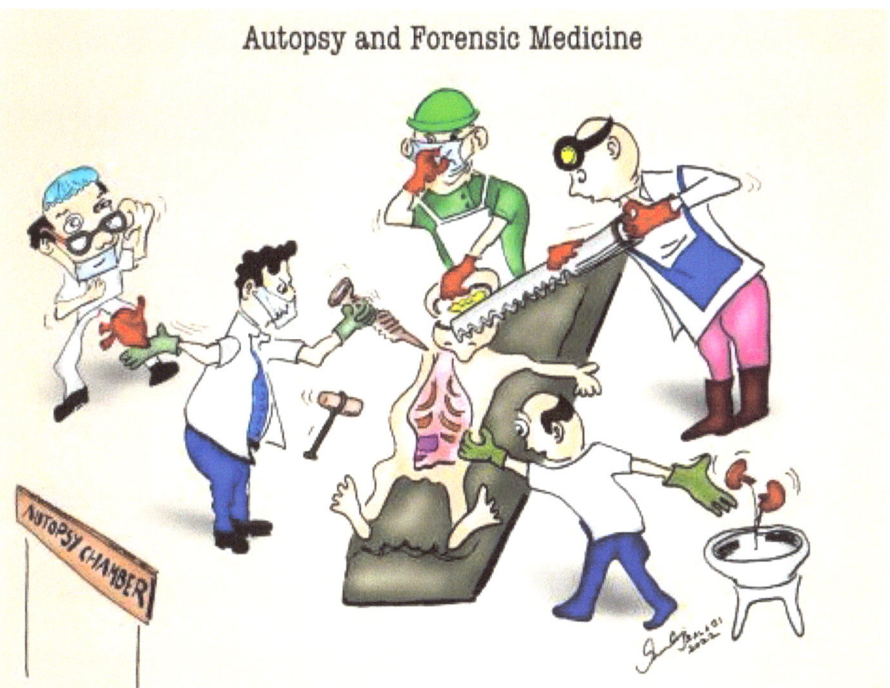

Figure 8.2: Autopsy and forensic medicine

8.2.7 Role of a Medical or Dental Officer

A dentist or medical professional has two jobs to do when faced with a person's apparent death. The first step in a death diagnosis is to proclaim the person dead once all signs of life have permanently vanished.

The second step is to determine and confirm the cause of death. The doctor fills out the "death report" as an informant after determining the patient is deceased. For each death, the legal information and statistical information fields of the death report must be completed. The medical certificate of cause of death (MCCD) and the death report (form 4) are sent to the Death Registry authority.

A certificate of cause of death should be issued by the same medical professional who announces the death. Natural deaths are those brought on by old age and any diseases or problems that develop spontaneously.

The medical officer completes the first duty, which is the pronouncement of death, if there are any questions about the cause of death or if the cause of death is unknown or uncertain (if it is not a natural death), and then tells the police of the death's occurrence for further action. A medical certificate of cause of death (MCCD) won't be issued by him.

In some situations, the cremation ground employees or municipality staff will not grant approval to cremate or bury the body, even if the families desire to, if the reason for death is not indicated on the form. If anybody tries to cremate the corpse without a valid death certificate and a cause of death determination, this is done to avoid foul play (when suspected of a criminal or a medico-legal death).

After the corpse is in the possession of the investigating officer, an inquest will be conducted, and the cause of death will be determined following the medical-legal postmortem. Ordinarily, the investigating officer, coroner, or magistrate issues the directive to do the medico-legal postmortem. The medical examiner who performs the postmortem or hospital officials will determine the cause of death when the autopsy is finished. The police will send the death reporting authority a copy of this autopsy

certificate along with the death report forms.

8.3 Guidelines for issuing MCCD

Along with the explanations provided above regarding certifications, the practitioner should also be aware of the following:

- As soon as he is certain of the cause of death, he shouldn't wait to issue the MCCD. He is not permitted to collect a fee for issuing this certificate.
- The physician should not certify the cause of death on the medical record before the patient has passed away or without personally inspecting and examining the corpse.
- Even if the families have not paid the doctor's debts, the doctor shall not delay issuing the medical certificate of cause of death.
- Although it is not legally obligatory, in some facilities, the medical supervisor should countersign the death report.
- The dead must have been seen by the doctor within seven days prior to death.
- If the death is not natural, the registrar may record the occasion of the death and indicate in the cause of death column that an inquest report is pending.

No MCCD shall be given, and the dead body should not be discharged if
- The wounded are brought dead.
- The cops have reported a crime. The matter has already been reported to the police. The cause of death is unknown.

8.3.1 How to fill out the MCCD (Medical Cause of Death Certificate)

There are two categories of death certificates:

1) Form 4: For fatalities that take place in hospitals
2) For non-institutional fatalities, use Form 4A.

They are different in that the Form 4 contains information on the hospital where the death happened, and the Form 4A contains information about the physician who treated the patient.

The WHO suggested two elements for the medical certificate of cause of death (form 4/4A) in order to simplify consistent reporting:

- Upper part: information on the dead is provided, along with medical information regarding the cause of death.
- Lower part: Details on the dead, together with the time, date, and location of the death.

Personal particulars of the deceased:
Name of the deceased: Be sure to include the middle name if it exists, as well as the first and last names (surname). There must be no initials. For newborns who have not yet been given names, write son or daughter of, followed by the names of the father and mother. Don't forget to mention the father's name as well (or the husband's name for a married female).

Write your age in years if you are older than a year. Enter in months and days if the child is under one year old.

8.3.2 Method of Certification of Death

Part I, Cause(s) of Death: Since the attending physician will be the only one to determine the cause of death, it is crucial that the physician properly document the cause of death. Gross inaccuracies in death data and their direct impact on national health policy and recommendations are caused by wrong diagnosis or improper certificate filling. In medico-legal matters, the MCCD may also be subject to judicial review. If the reason for death is incorrectly recorded, it could not stand up under interrogation in court. The competency of the granting authority is therefore questioned.

Due to incompetence or apathy, doctors sometimes make serious errors when determining the cause of death. It is quite regrettable that this topic is not given significant weight in the medical and dentistry school curricula. According to data from several sources, 50 to 60 percent of MCCDs are incorrectly filled. This is a significant worry that might have equally catastrophic repercussions.

Dental surgeons must get training in the methods and steps involved in issuing MCCDs and pronouncing death. Although the Dental Council of India (DCI) advises that the certificate should only be given to a patient who has been treated by them or is under their supervision, it is crucial to explain the death and determine the reason for it.

The dentist or any other dental specialist must be fully aware of the patient's medical history because dental surgeons may not be engaged in the general well-being and treatments that a patient receives. This can be discovered by looking through the patient's medical records and conducting an examination. Appropriate certification depends on knowing a patient's medical history.

The doctor who treated the patient will determine the time and date of death, which must be included in the first section of the form. Any death following dental treatment, whether outside the boundaries of the dental office or at home, shall be the moment at which another physician first meets the patient, regardless of the time of death, as the attending physician cannot verify the time of death without viewing the patient. For instance, the exact moment of death should be reported as the time at which the patient was discovered dead if they had an extraction or other minor surgical treatment, went home, and subsequently passed away.

When determining the cause of death, knowledge about the patient's medical history and co-existing illnesses is extremely beneficial. It is advised that you see your family doctor in this respect.

The death certificate can only be completed following an autopsy in cases of suicide attempts due to psychosocial problems or motor vehicle accidents, and certification completion will be carried out in collaboration with the pathologists from forensic medicine and/or the agencies conducting the investigation before the MCCD is given to the registrar of births and deaths of state governments. It is noteworthy that some unnatural deaths, such as suicide, can happen after receiving medical or surgical care. This includes passing away from despair brought on by a poor diagnosis or being unhappy with the results of surgery. [3]

These are unique situations that require consideration as unnatural deaths. In order to comply with medico-legal requirements, it is also the hospital's duty to notify the police if a suspicious death happens there. The corpse of the deceased shall be given over for forensic and medicolegal inquiry in all situations where the reason for death is unknown in order to determine the accurate reason for death by postmortem. The cause of death is determined during a postmortem study in cases where a patient passes away following outpatient dental or maxillofacial surgery. The inquest and post-mortem examination results will be used to determine the lawful time of death. However, if a patient experiences a complication that necessitates numerous attempts at resuscitation, the moment of death should be reported as soon as those efforts are abandoned as fruitless.

If a patient dies in the hospital, certain medical facilities have a policy of keeping the body for two hours to check for signs of life. This is to ensure that death is not misdiagnosed, and in such cases, the attending physician will determine the time of death. Any personal data should be reported as 'unknown' until the proper information and identification are accessible if a death happens to an unidentified individual following dental treatment ***Cause of Death***:

> In 1967, the World Health Assembly designated "all those diseases, morbid conditions, or harm that ultimately resulted in death or contributed to death, and the conditions of accident or violence that caused any such injuries" as the causes of death.

Each line should ideally include one cause. Events that lead to death should be the subject of the second line. In the final line, you should include the underlying cause of death. They outline the series of circumstances that, if accurately recorded, ultimately resulted in death. For instance, if a person dies from significant bleeding while sitting in a dentist's chair, the death will be documented as

- *Line Ia: Immediate cause of death*: shock
- *Line Ib: Antecedent cause*: hypotension from acute and severe bleeding
- *Line Ic: Underlying cause*: Not known (underlying bleeding disorder)

Line (Ia) is always used to report the immediate cause. This is the illness, injury, or complication that happened before the person died. It is required that you enter that information on I (a). Death modes like post-operative bleeding or respiratory failure shouldn't even be included because they are more symptoms than actual causes of death. This includes the patient who died from a violent death, like a severe head injury associated with maxillofacial injuries.

Line (Ib): consequence of an underlying disease; for example, a patient had a recent history of myocardial infarction and died in the dental office because of ventricular tachycardia, ventricular fibrillation, or cardiac asystole. That must be written in the second line. So, if a patient who died had an RTA and a head injury, the sequence in (b) should be a fracture of the skull.

Line (Ic): The underlying cause should be the one that gives rise to the antecedent cause. For example, a dead patient was under the influence of alcohol at the time of the accident, and it must be entered in line (I c).

Part II: Other significant conditions:
The purpose of Section II of the death certificate is to include all other illnesses or ailments that are thought to have negatively impacted the progress of the morbid process and hence contributed to the overall outcome, in order of significance. They are connected to the illness or condition that is the direct cause of mortality.

The death certificate must list any medical issues that the deceased person had that were directly connected to the reason for death, such as a previous myocardial infarction, since they may have contributed to their demise.

The coexisting illness shouldn't be listed as the underlying cause of death on the death certificate if it is unlikely to have been the cause of death.

It is significant to highlight that the patient's illnesses may not have all been connected in any manner to the cause of death.

It is important to write the names of the illnesses clearly and completely. Avoid using illness abbreviations and abbreviated forms. When expressing the sequence of events, one must avoid using ambiguous, insufficient phrases and descriptions that are similarly poor. Similar to this, symptomatic comments have no place on a certificate.

A format endorsed by the WHO should be used to document the cause of death. The root cause of death, the antecedent cause of death, and the proximate cause of death are all clearly shown from below upwards on a properly filled certificate under Section I. According to time and etio-pathological relationships, the recorded events should be in chronological order and be related to one another.

The significance of the order of occurrences is to highlight any potential advantages of involvement and to aid in making judgements in similar situations in the future.

According to the 43rd World Health Assembly's recommendations in 1990, additional lines (d, e) can be added to the original WHO form to describe the order in which the causes of death occurred. This is stated on page 17 of the WHO document, Medical Certification of Causes of Death.

Female death: Even though pregnancy had nothing to do with the death, information on pregnancy is required in the event that a woman receiving dental or surgical care of childbearing age (15–49 years) passes away. This demonstrates how crucial it is for dentists to be aware of women's pregnant status, especially after marriage, in order to protect the interests of safe operations and prevent undesired medical and legal complications in the event that a patient dies as a result of any dental-related procedures.

Child death: The complete sequence must be properly stated on the death certificate if a newborn dies in a dentist office or other relevant circumstances. Before performing any surgical or dental operations, the practitioner must obtain a comprehensive history of the case from the patient's parents or records. This is crucial for kids with congenital abnormalities, such as heart defects, in particular. [3]

At this stage, it's important to keep in mind that children with craniofacial diseases frequently have heart defects. This is due to the fact that the growth of the face and heart both occur at the same time and are impacted by inappropriate neural crest cell migration, resulting in syndromic newborns with both cardiac and facial defects.

Compared to typical newborns, they are more likely to have morbidity from dental or maxillofacial treatments carried out under local or general anesthesia. Children. Additionally, they might be born with other significant metabolic flaws.

The majority of death certificates will additionally stipulate that the deceased's epidemiological data be included.

8.3.3 Certifier Details (Details Regarding the Doctor)

The certifier signs the death certificate after filling out parts I and II with all pertinent information, including the cause of death, and after providing his name, credentials, designation, and registration number. Except in circumstances where the reason for death has been established following an autopsy, the time and date of signing should match those provided at the commencement of the certificate. The certificate must be stamped with the hospital's official seal or the involved practitioner's clinic seal.

Certificate to relatives:
When there is a lower part, the relatives receive it. It contains information about the dead as well as the date, time, and location of the death. This will assist them in gaining municipal authorities' approval for cremation and serve as a registry for requesting a summary of the death register (death certificate) from the registration authority. It could be wise to bring out at this stage that the part sent to family members might not include the reason for death. According to Section 17(1)(b) of the Registration of Birth and

Death Act of 1969, this will maintain the confidentiality of information regarding the cause of death.

8.3.4 Handing Over the Certificate to the Registering Authority

The hospital or qualified practitioner (in the event of dental office certification) must give the registering authority the death certificate directly within a time frame of 7 to 14 days. The registration authority's register should contain a record of the medical reason. Section 17(1)(b) of the Act forbids sending certifications through relatives for the convenience and comfort of the hospital or the certifier.

8.3.5 Medical Certificate of Cause of Death[8]

It is necessary to have a template of examples to aid in the correct filling up of the cause of death, especially in the area of dentistry and maxillofacial services, where so far, no vital statistics have been given by the Registrar General of India, although the DCI code of ethics regulation requires a registered dental surgeon to resuscitate and treat emergency cases, declare death, and certify the cause.

The following are some guidelines for filling up pertinent details to be written in the cause of death columns corresponding to the major cause group of mortality:

1. **Infections:** acute, sub-acute, or chronic infections in the maxillofacial area leading to death. The name of the disease, like Ludwig's angina; the site, if localised or spreading; the method of transmission; and fascial space involvement, if relevant.

2. **Neoplasms:** morphological and histopathological type—whatever is known, whether it was benign or malignant; site of origin of primary growth in the maxillofacial area and metastasis to the chest or other organs; or whether the primary lesion is somewhere else in the body and metastasis is to the facial bones, etc.

3. **Endocrine disorders:** type of disease, process, or function in any gland An example patient died due to adrenaline in local anaesthesia, precipitating a thyroid crisis (toxic) or in a patient with an adrenal crisis due to long-term steroid intake, leading to other complications like adrenal insufficiency and hypotension.

4. **Blood disorders:** nature of disease and type of deficiency; example: bleeding disorders, whether hereditary or acquired Underlying central vascular malformations in the maxillofacial skeleton, etc.

5. **Nervous system disorders:** uncontrolled or precipitated epilepsy during a dental procedure Pre-existing known disease under medication. Motor neuron disease, parkinsonism with stridor, etc. are other examples.

6. **Circulatory diseases:** nature of disease, acute or chronic where relevant; aetiology, like infective endocarditis from rheumatic heart disease; myocardial infarction during dental procedures or postoperative death; secondary cardiac complications after major maxillofacial surgery.

7. **Respiratory diseases:** nature of disease, acute or chronic; like asthmatics and associated

complications in dental chairs leading to mortality.

8. **Congenital disorders:** size and type of complications; type of cranial and other syndrome abnormalities like raised ICP, etc.

9. **Musculoskeletal disorders:** nature of the disease process; any infective organism; underlying diseases; type size; and whether there are any congenital or acquired deformities.

10. **Adverse effects of drugs in therapeutic use:** for example, anaphylaxis after a dental prescription. State this fact and the name of the drug, the nature of the adverse effect, complications, and conditions treated.

11. **Anaesthetic causes:** airway disease, compromised type of anaesthesia, postoperative issues in the ICU, etc.

12. **Foreign body aspiration:** type of foreign body lost in the pharynx in a dental chair, measures taken to remove it, initial resuscitation attempts, etc.

Examples of certification

Though many examples of medical certification have been illustrated and explained in the bulletin of the Office of the Registrar General of India (Ministry of Home Affairs), so far no textbook or manual has given any clear-cut guidelines for maxillofacial surgeons and dental surgeons regarding the examples of certification in their field.

Annexure 1 (Form No. 2): Death report consisting of Legal information which has to be added to the Death Register and Statistical information which has to be detached and sent for statistical processing

FORM NO.2 (See Rule 5)	DEATH REPORT Legal information *This part to be added to the Death Register*		DEATH REPORT Statistical information This part to be detached and sent for statistical processing	FORM NO.2 (See Rule 5)
To be filled by the informant		*To be filled by the informant*	*To be filled by the informant*	
1.	**Date of Death** : (Enter the exact day, month and year the child was born e.g. 1-1-2000)	11.	**Town or Village of Residence of the deceased** : (Place where the deceased actually lived. This can be different from the place where the death occurred. The house address is not required to be entered.) a) **Name of Town/Village :** b) **Is it a town or village :** (Tick the appropriate entry below) **1. Town 2. Village** c) **Name of District :** d) **Name of State :**	15.	**Was the cause of death medically certified?:** (Tick the appropriate entry below) 1. Yes . 2. No
2.	Name of the Deceased : (Full name as usually written) UID No of Father (if any)			16.	**Name of Disease or Actual Cause of Death** : (For all deaths irrespective of whether medically certified or not)
3.	Sex of the deceased : (Enter "Male" or "Female"or "Transgender") Do not use abbreviation)	12.	**Religion :** (Tick the appropriate entry below) **1.Hindu 2. Muslim 3.Christian** **4. Any other religion :** (write name of the religion)	17.	**In case this is a female death, did the death occur while pregnant, at the time of delivery or within 6 weeks after the end of pregnancy:** (Tick the appropriate entry below) **1.Yes 2. No**
4.	Name of the Mother : UID No of Father (if any)				
5.	Name of the Father : UID No of Mother (if nay)	13.	**Occupation of the deceased:** (If no occupation write 'Nil')	18.	**If used to habitually smoke – for how many years?**
5a	Name of the Husband / Wife : UID No of Mother (if nay)	14.	*Type of medical attention received before death:* *(Tick the appropriate entry below)* *1. Institutional* *2. Medical attention other than institution* *3. No medical attention*	19.	**If used to habitually chew tobacco in any form – for how many years?**
6.	**Age of the deceased :** (If the deceased was over 1 year of age, give age in completed years. If the deceased was below 1 year of age, give age in months, and if below 1 month give age in completed number of days, and if below one day, in hours)				
7.	Address of the deceased at the time of Death:				
8.	Permanent address of the deceased: Mobile No :			20.	**If used to habitually chew arecanut in any form (including pan masala) – for how many years?**
9	Place of death: (Tick the appropriate entry 1,2 or 3 below and give the name of the Hospital/Institution or the address of the house where the death took place, If other place give location) 1.Hospital/ Institution Name & Address: 2.House Address : 3. Others:			21.	**If used to habitually drink alcohol – for how many years?**
10	Informant's name : Address : *(After completing* *All columns 1 to 21,* *Informant will put* *date and signature here :)*				
Date : **Signature or left thumb mark of the informant**			*(Columns to be filled are over. Now put signature at left)*	
To be filled by the Registrar			*To be filled by the Registrar*	
Registration No: Registration date : Registration Unit : Town/Village : District : Remarks (If any) Name and Signature of the Registrar		District : Tahsil : Town / Village : Registration Unit :	Name	Code No.	Registration No: Registration date : Date of Death : Sex : 1.Male 2.Female Age : Years / Months/Days / Hours Place of Death: 1.Hospital / Institution 2. House Name and Signature of the Registrar

To be detached and sent for statistical Processing

Annexure 2 (Form No. 6): Death Certificate

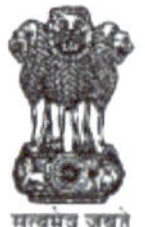

प्ररूप सं. 6

FORM NO. 6

मृत्यु प्रमाण–पत्र

DEATH CERTIFICATE

(जन्म और मृत्यु रजिस्ट्रीकरण अधिनियम, 1969 की धारा 12/17 और

राजस्थान जन्म और मृत्यु रजिस्ट्रीकरण नियम, 2000 के नियम 8/13 के अधीन जारी किया गया)

(Issued under Section 12/17 of the Registration of Births and Deaths Act,1969 and Rule 8/13 of the Rajasthan Registration of Births and Deaths Rules, 2000)

यह प्रमाणित किया जाता है कि निम्न लिखित सूचना मृत्यु के मूल अभिलेख से ली गई है जो कि (स्थानीय क्षेत्र/स्थानीय निकाय) ....

.... तहसील /खण्ड.. जिला ....राज्य../संघ राज्य

क्षेत्र ....का रजिस्टर है।

This is to certify that the following information has been taken from the original record of death which is the register for (local area / local body)...............................of tahsil / block........................... of District...................................of state / Union territory ....

नाम/Name: ....लिंग/ Sex .... मृत्यु

की तिथि/Date of Death ....मृत्यु स्थान /Place of death........................... माता का

नाम/Name of mother...

पिता/पति का नाम / Name of Father/Husband ....

<table>
<tr><td>मृतक का मृत्यु के समय का पता</td><td>मृतक का स्थायी पता</td></tr>
<tr><td>Address of the deceased at the time of death:</td><td>Permanent address of the deceased:</td></tr>
</table>

....

....

....

रजिस्ट्रीकरण सं../Registration No:. .... रजिस्ट्रीकरण की तारीख / Date of Registration ....

टिप्पणी/Remarks(if any)..

जारी करने की तारीख / Date of issue:.................................जारी करने वाले प्राधिकारी के हस्ताक्षर/Signature of the issuing authority

जारी करने वाले प्राधिकारी का पता / Address of the issuing authority

मुहर /Seal

Annexure 3 (Form 4A): Medical Certificate of cause of death (For non-Institutional death. No to be used for still births)

<u>**FORM NO. 4A**</u>
(See Rule 7)
<u>**MEDICAL CERTIFICATE OF CAUSE OF DEATH**</u>
(For non-institutional deaths. Not to be used for still births)
To be sent to Registrar along with Form No. 2 (Death Report)

I hereby certify that the deceased Shri/Smt/Km……………………………………………… son/wife/daughter of …………………………………… resident of ……………………………………………………… was under my treatment from ……………………… to ………………………… and he/she died on ……………………………… at ………………A.M./P.M.

NAME OF DECEASED					For use of Statistical Office
Sex	Age at Death				
	If 1 year or more, age in years	If less than 1 year, age in month	If less than one month, age in days	If less than one day, age in hours	
3. Male 4. Female					

<u>**CAUSE OF DEATH**</u>		Interval between onset and death approx.
I Immediate cause State the disease, injury or complication which caused death, not the mode of dying such as heart failure, asthenia, etc.	(a) …………………………………… due to (or as a consequences of)	
Antecedent cause Morbid conditions, if any, giving rise to the above cause, stating underlying conditions last	(b) …………………………………… due to (or as a consequences of)	
II Other significant conditions contributing to the death but not related to the disease or condition causing it	(c) …………………………………… …………………………………… ……………………………………	

If deceased was a female, was pregnancy the death associated with?   1. Yes 2. No
If yes, was there a delivery?   1. Yes   2. No

Name and signature of the Medical Practitioner certifying the cause of death

Date of verification ………………………………………………………………………

SEE REVERSE FOR INSTRUCTIONS

(To be detached and handed over to the relative of the deceased)

Certified that Shri/Smt/Kum……………………………………... S/W/D of Shri …………………………………………..

R/O ……………………………………………. was under my treatment from …………………………………

to ……………………………… and he/she expired on ………………………………………… at ………………… A.M./P.M.

Doctor …………………………………………………..
Signature and address of Medical Practitioner/
Medical attendant with Registration No.

Annexure 4: Medical Certificate of cause of death (Hospital In-patients. Not to be used for still births)

FORM NO. 4

(See Rule 7)

MEDICAL CERTIFICATE OF CAUSE OF DEATH

(Hospital in-patients. Not to be used for still births)

To be sent to Registrar along with Form No. 2 (Death Report)

Name of the Hospital   …………………………………................………………..

I hereby certify that the person whose particulars are given below died in the hospital in Ward No. ………. On at ………. AM/PM.

NAME OF DECEASED					
Sex	Age at Death				For use of Statistical Office
	If 1 year or more, age in years	If less than 1 year, age in months	If less than one month, age in Days	If less than one day, age in Hours	
1. Male 2. Female					
CAUSE OF DEATH				Interval between on set & death approx.	
I. **Immediate cause** State the disease, injury or complication which caused death, not the mode of dying such as heart failure, asthenia etc.			(a)……………………………………… …………….. Due to (or as a consequences of)		
Antecedent cause Morbid conditions, if any, giving rise to the above Cause, stating underlying condition last			(b)……………………………………… ………………….. Due to (or as a consequences of)		
II Other significant conditions contributing to the death but not related to the disease or conditions causing II			© ……………………………………………… ………………… ………………………………………………		

Manner of Death   How did the injury occur?

1. Natural   2. Accident   3. Suicide   4. Homicide

5. Pending Investigation

If deceased was a female, was pregnancy the death associated with? 1. Yes 2. No

If yes, was there a delivery? 1. Yes 2. No

Name and signature of the Medical Attendant certifying the cause of death

Date of verification ……………………………………………

___

(To be detached and handed over to the related of the deceased)

Certified that Shri/Smt/Km ……………………..S/W/D of Shri. …………………..

R/O ………………………was admitted to this hospital on …….. and expired on

……………………………………..

Doctor ……………….

(Medical Supdt.

Name of Hospital

8.4 Conclusion

The dental professional or any doctor who fulfils the task of writing a death certificate and identifying the reason or causes of death has a responsibility to provide accurate and thorough certification. A thorough understanding of the pathophysiology of the fundamental causes of death and potential factors that contribute to death aids in handling this task with confidence and competence. It is entirely conceivable that numerous questions and clarifications may arise when filling out the form. This establishes the veracity of the certifier's claim that the death certificate has been prepared "to the best of my knowledge!" while signing it.

The Army Directive 1/2003/MP recommends that death certificates be provided following a post-mortem and in conjunction with the divisional medical officer or given to the local civil police authority in cases involving the army and fatalities in dentistry practice. Before giving the document to the registering authority, Army Headquarters (AHQ) may append a separate page with all the regimental officer's information if necessary. The form required for death declaration in the army is AFMSF 93 part, which contains all the pertinent information indicated in this chapter, including the cause of death. However, it may not be required, as all cases may undergo a postmortem before the final certificate is handed over.

References:

1. Commonwealth of Pennsylvania, Department of Health, Bureau of Health Statistics & Research, 2012 Death Certificate Registration Manual Revised December 28, 2011

2. Tamil nadu registration of births and deaths rules 2000 (G.O.Ms. No. 528, Health and Family Welfare (AB-2), 29th December 1999). **http://cms. tn.gov.in/sites/default/files/rules/ birth_ death_rules_e.pdf/**

3. Medical Examiners' and Coroners' handbook on death registration and fetal death reporting 2003 Revision, Maryland DHHS publication.

4. Swapnil S. Agarwal et al. Medical certification of cause of death. J Indian Acad Forensic Med, 30(4).

5. The registration of births and deaths act, 1969 (Act no. 18 of 1969). www. pbnrhm.org/ docs/b&d_reg.pdf

6. Dental council of India notification **www.wbja.nic.in/../** **The** revised dental Reg.ul 4, 2014

7. The registration (births and deaths act) http://moj.gov.jm/sites/default/ files/laws/

8. O.p. Murty et al. Uniform guidelines for postmortem work in india: faculty development on standard operative Procedures (sop) in forensic medicine and toxicology. Journal of forensic medicine & toxicology vol. 30 no. 1 & 2, january - december 2013

Death in Dental Chair / Hospital During Procedures

9.1 Introduction

Though it is very difficult to answer this question of mortality related procedures in one word, we can simply say that by following the protocol that we have described in this book, most questions will be answered. Once the death occurs in a dental practice or hospital where the patient is under the care of a consultant dentist or maxillofacial surgeon, the primary responsibility of initial post-death care management lies in the hands of a dentist or surgeon if one decides to declare the patient dead.

It is of paramount importance that the death be confirmed by the dental specialist by means of assessing certain signs of death as early as possible. At this juncture, the dentist may doubt whether the patient should be transferred to a hospital for a declaration of death. We wish to stress the fact that if a dentist is able to declare death on the basis of the clinical findings as explained in this book, he/she need not shift the patient to another hospital and seek the help of another physician to declare death.

But if there is a possibility of even a remote chance of life on clinical examination, the patient must be transported to the neighbouring medical centre for appropriate medical treatment as soon as possible without discussion or wasting time on unnecessary investigations within the clinic itself. Once the patient slips into a coma or nearing death stage due to shock or myocardial infarction, every minute matters, and, as a health service provider, it is the responsibility of the attending dentist or surgeon to move the patient into a quality medical care centre so that every chance is given to save the life of the patient.

Many of the medico-legal cases relating to death have been settled outside the court, as the relatives sometimes understand the gravity of the situation and also feel satisfied with the responsibility and action taken by the dentist or surgeon prior to death. This *"out of court settlement"* is possible if the relatives concerned are convinced of the terms of the dental or maxillofacial surgeon concerned.

Once death happens in dental practice or in a hospital set up, it is a grave matter for all the parties concerned, including relatives as well as the dental specialist team. Unless a surgeon or dentist knows how to handle the situation, this may be a challenging phase if there are any accusations regarding the procedure. It is important to note that any unnatural death, even in a dental clinic or waiting area or after a patient goes home after a procedure, must be autopsied to avoid any future medico-legal implications and also to know what could have been the possible cause of death.

9.2 Reasons for Death in the Dental Office

Most dental treatments are non-emergency and are done on an outpatient basis, and those cases that are reported for health emergencies in a dental office are mostly due to underlying medical problems or, rarely, as a complication of the dental treatment of both adult and paediatric patients.

The following list of reasons may be the cause of death, and its autopsy protocols are summarized below[1]:

- Myocardial Infarction: blood investigation, ECG if available, C9 immunochemistry, Cardiac marker examination: troponin, the diagnosis is aided by a thorough macroscopic and histological examination of the heart.
- Intracranial bleed (stroke) *in* severe hypertension patients following extraction
- Extraction *bleeding*—caused by underlying central haemangioma
- Aspiration *of* dentures, endodontic files, and crowns
- Endocrine problems—adrenal crisis; thyroid crisis—examined by studying the adrenal and thyroid glands
- Severe infections, Ludwig's angina
- Drug overdose, L.A toxicity/Sedation
- Airway obstruction from aspiration, pneumonia, or foreign body aspiration

9.3 Reasons for Death in Oral and Maxillofacial Surgery

Severe Craniofacial or head injury
- If accessible, the Glasgow Scale, X-ray, CT scan, and MRI of the deceased should be used to properly assess the severity.
- Less than 8 on the Glasgow coma scale indicates significant harm. Opening the skull and seeing into the brain during an autopsy is the only way to record the results since they can be either under- or over-reported.
- Since linear fractures are difficult to see in photographs, skull fractures should also be depicted using sketch diagrams.
- Damage to the intracranial contents continues to be the leading traumatic cause of death.
- Blood collections of over 70 mL have significant pressure consequences. The brain's maximum adjusting capacity is between 150 and 200 ml, which has a quick death rate.
- Due to pressure necrosis, herniation sites such as the cerebellar tonsils, parahippocampal gyrus, and uncal region may appear black or discoloured and will have a pronounced depression of bony projections. These have to be photographed, and a histological inspection of the sections is also instructive.
- A base haemorrhage of greater than 30 ml results in death. Any pontine haemorrhage larger than the size of a huge pinhead is nearly always deadly.

- The combination of subdural and subarachnoid haemorrhages is most frequently encountered in head injury situations.
- Additionally, notable findings in these instances include contusions and diffuse axonal damage.

Neck: carotid injury; fat or air embolism:
- During neck dissection, carotid bleed can occur due to accidental damage, leading to blood loss and death.
- Check for air bubbles in the great veins and epicardial arteries.
- Fat embolism occurs especially in limb injuries, and air embolisms occur due to head and neck injuries in RTA.
- Hemo-pneumothrorax: due to chest injuries or rib fractures.
- Cor pulmonale: cardiac examination done to assess right ventricular hypertrophy and sizes of pulmonary artery; evaluation of BNP (Brain natriuretic peptide) in blood

Blood loss. Bleed- in peritoneum, iliac injuries result in shock and death.

　GA/ LA complication - The majority of the time, they happen during surgery or just after the surgical procedure

9.4 Classification of Deaths Associated with Invasive Procedures and Anaesthesia

1. Those brought on directly by the illness or damage that the invasive treatment or anaesthesia was being utilised to treat.
2. Those brought on by a sickness or condition unrelated to the one for which the surgery was carried out.
3. Those brought on by an error made during or a problem with the invasive technique.
4. Those brought on by an error in the application of an anaesthetic or as a result of a related problem.

9.5 Common Fatal Complications of Invasive Procedures

Bronchopneumonia, multi-organ failure, pulmonary embolism, peri-operative myocardial infarction, haemorrhage, and sepsis.

9.5.1 Anaesthetic Deaths

Sensitivity, hypotension, and cardiac ischemia during the induction phase
- Instrumentation: oxygen cylinders, gas connections, and tube integrity mishaps.
- Electricity: defective equipment and current leaks
- 'Faulty intubation'
- Aspiration of gastric contents.
- Negligence: throat pack or gauze left in situ, bleeding from the nose during nasotracheal intubation, compromised airway patients, including use of sedatives in such groups
- Dislodgements of broken dentures, orthodontic brackets or wires, and crowns, reamers, endodontic files and fractured teeth into orotracheal region during intubation.

Anaesthesia-related death can be divided into four parts:
1. Preoperative period: excessive sedation and medication

2. Beginning (induction phase): producing anaesthesia, inadequate sensitization
3. Long operations throughout the surgery necessitated high dosages.
4. Post-operative

9.6 Important Points If a Death or Near Death Happens in the Dental Chair or a Hospital

(Figure 9.1)

1. The first and foremost is not to panic and create confusion among your team and relatives of the patient.
2. Call for help from nearby assistants if available, or call (can be made by the clinic assistant or receptionist) for an ambulance if chances of life exist after primary treatment.
3. Regain your composure, and quietly and swiftly review the situation and make sure that all possible measures and treatments have been taken before one concludes that life has ceased for the patient.
4. If a dental specialist feels that there is a possibility of life, then move the patient immediately to a nearby hospital.
5. If no signs of life are observed, inform the relatives quietly and boldly that an incident has occurred.
6. Inform the police about the incident immediately and ask for help for further proceedings. Do not remove anything used during the procedure and resuscitation from the room until police personnel arrive and assume control of the proceedings.
7. Do not try to remove any crucial evidence that may be useful for your defence in court.
8. Speak to the relatives, appraise them of the situation, and an opinion can be sought from the police on the protocol to be followed.
9. Kindly refrain from obstruction if the patient's relatives want an autopsy for legal purposes and for the purpose of confirmation of death.
10. Help the relatives arrange for transportation for the autopsy if need arises to alleviate any suspicion by the patient's family towards yourself as culpable in the death.
11. If you have case records in the clinic, complete them correctly by describing the entire event from the start of the procedure.
12. Specifically mention in the notes the type of drug used (with the correct dosage) for lifesaving and the equipment used for resuscitation with O_2 facility if it was available.
13. If your clinic has a video surveillance facility, it may be useful evidence in court when a patient's relatives accuse you of any inaction in the clinic.
14. But if a patient is not interested in an autopsy, the question will be whether to send the deceased patient for an autopsy or not. [2-4]

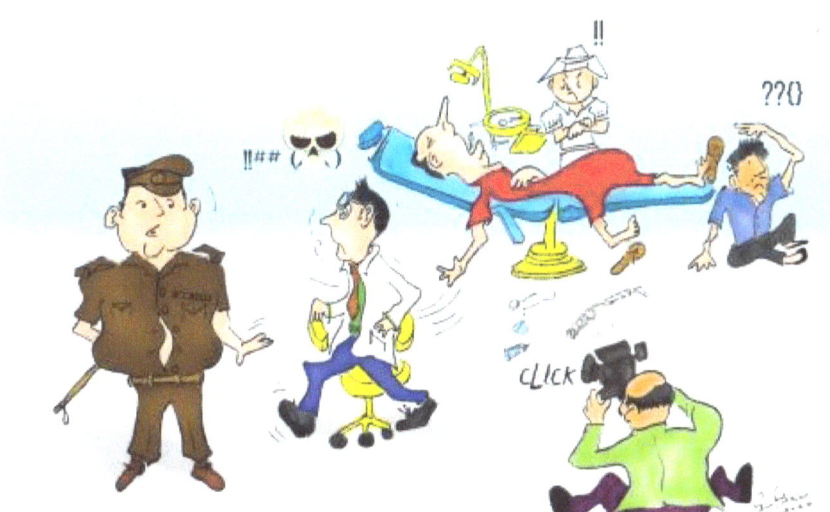

Figure 9.1: In the event of death in dental chair

References

1. Coplans MP, Curson I. Deaths associated with dentistry and dental disease 1980–1989. Anaesthesia. 1993 May;48(5):435-8.

2. Correspondence. Death in the dental chair. Anaesthesia, 1999, 54, pages 703–721

3. L.M.Worthington et al. death in dental chair: an avoidable catastrophe?. British journal of anaesthesia. Vol 80, No.2. Feb 1998

4. Helen H. Lee et al. Trends in Death Associated with Pediatric Dental Sedation and General Anesthesia. Paediatr Anaesth. 2013 August; 23(8): 741–746. doi:10.1111/pan.12210.

Role of Dental Records for Death Certification and in Court of Law for Alleged Malpractice

After the death of a patient, in order to counter any alleged malpractice against the dental surgeons the dental records play a vital role in court of law if warranted.

The dental record, also referred to as the patient's chart, is the official office document that records all of the treatment done and all patient-related communications that occur in the dental office. The dental record provides for continuity of care for the patient and is critical in the event of a malpractice insurance claim.

10.1. Importance of Records

These records should contain all diagnostic information, clinical notes, treatment performed and patient-related communications that occur in the dental office, including instructions for home care and consent to treatment. At the same time the confidentiality of the patient's dental and medical health status should be maintained.

Diligent and complete record keeping is extremely important for many reasons.
First, it can contribute to providing the best possible **care for the patient**. Patient records document the course of treatment and may provide data that can be used in evaluating the quality of care that is provided to the patient.

Records also provide a **means of communication** between the treating dentist and any other doctor who will care for that patient. Complete and accurate records contain enough information to allow another dental or medical provider who has no prior knowledge of the patient to know the patient's dental experience in your office. In the unfortunate death of an outpatient dental clinic treated by us in a neighboring hospital where the patient self-referred there before death, the hospital authorities may ask for records pertinent to dental treatment done and if not satisfactory information given alleged malpractice can arise.

Beyond providing patient care, the dental record is important because it may be used in a court of law to establish the diagnostic information that was obtained and the treatment that was rendered to the patient prior to the death. For example, if emergency drugs were available in the clinic, drugs used, resuscitation techniques performed etc. The records can also be used in **defense of allegations of malpractice**. Information found in the record may then be used in determining whether the diagnosis and treatment conformed to the standards of care expected as per the guidelines of dental council of India.

Though not directly related to death of a dental patient, records will help to provide information to appropriate legal authorities that will **aid in the identification of a dead or missing person**. This is particularly important if a dental patient who had treatment goes outside state or a country and then found dead, the dental treatment of the diseased person may be sought after for records for mistaken identity and medico-legal forensic (forensic dentistry) purposes.

10.2. Organization of Dental Records

Most dentists make notes in paper dental records. However, more and more dentists are making use of computerized filling systems to maintain patient dental records. Electronic records have great quality and patient-safety benefits, and will likely increase as more dental offices become computerized. Because many dental offices use the traditional paper charts, traditional filing systems are discussed first.

Generally, patient records are housed in file folders for protection. These files are labeled with the following information (in the following order):
- Patient's surname;
- Patient's first name;
- Patient's middle name if any available
- Patient's degree or seniority

The files are then arranged in a way for easy retrieval—usually in a lateral, open-shelf filing system.

Color Coding
Many dental offices use a color-coded filing system for patient record files. Color-coded labels usually the first two letters of the patient's last name and active date of treatment—are placed on the patient's file. This can help make record retrieval fast and easy.

Active and Inactive
Most offices have two categories of patient records files: 1) Active and 2) Inactive.

Active files hold the records of patients currently having their dental care provided by the practice.

Inactive patients are considered to be those who have not returned for 24 months. Keep files of active patients on-site. These records should be conveniently located in the office as backups.

Inactive files hold the records of patients who have been treated in the office in the past but are not currently under care in the office. These files are generally located in the office, but in a remote area.

For example in USA this is defined by policy of the American Dental Association, (Trans. 1991:621), an active dental patient of record is any individual in either of the following two categories: Category I - patients of record who have had dental service(s) provided by the dentist in the past twelve (12) months; Category II patients of record who have had dental service(s) provided by the dentist in the past twenty four (24) months, but not within the past twelve (12) months. An inactive patient is any individual who has become a patient of record and has not received any dental services(s) by the dentists in the past twenty-four (24) months. This system is not mandatory in all Indian clinics but can be used as a guide for future record maintenance in any dental clinic and dental hospital practice.

Though India state system does not have similar policy of the legal record maintenance, many established outpatient dental clinics and maxillofacial hospitals have electronic or conventional record maintenance practice which if full proof should be legibly written, all events relating to treatment and resuscitation of a patient if attempted before death.

All records, active and inactive, should be maintained carefully to be certain that they are not destroyed or lost as Indian legal system may take years to complete legal formality and completion hearing and judgment.

<h2>10.3 Content of the Dental Record</h2>

The information in the dental record should primarily be clinical in nature. The record includes a patient's registration form with all the basic personal information.

The dental team should be very meticulous and thorough in the dental office record keeping tasks. All information in the dental record should be clearly written, and the person / clinician responsible for entering new information should sign and date the entry. The information should not be ambiguous or contain many abbreviations. In practices with more than one dental practitioner, the identity of the practitioner rendering the treatment should be clearly noted in the record.

All entries in the patient record should be dated, initialed and handwritten in ink and/or computer printed. While no specific color of ink is required, (though many clinicians prefer **black ink** as it will legible for photocopying and scanning records for medico-legal purposes) any copy of the record should be easy to read. Handwritten entries should be legible. If a mistake is made, do not correct it with *"white-out."* A single line should be drawn through the incorrect info, the new corrected info added, and again, the entry should be signed and dated.

Importance of Writing the date and time of every action / Procedure done by a dentist or surgeon:

In the authors experience with a case of mortality in post-maxillofacial surgery, it was found that the timing was incorrect between the sequence events of written in the notes by different specialists. It was a case of a death in ICU due to drug reactions and an expert of anesthetists and pediatricians etc. investigated the whole event.

- Questions were raised on the drug history,
- Dosage of drug given for the weight of that patient
- Why there is an overwriting and change of drug dosage correction in the drug chart after the death of the patient. Automatically this raises suspicion on doctors and hospital records manipulation.

Specifically mention, the timings of event from

- What time the operation completed?
- Was there is any delay in recovery?
- What time the patient was shifted in ICU?
- What time the drug was given?
- Whether Oxygen and ECG monitors were present in ICU?
- Was there an intensivist / anesthetist covering the ICU?
- What time the doctor / ICU sister noticed respiratory arrest etc.

By going through all events, the enquiry committee felt that there is a total incoordination of events in timings written by surgeons, ICU in charge and anesthetist who declared the patient after a failed resuscitation attempt.

In the court of law this will be major embarrassment for the clinician and the lawyer to defend the sequence causes leading of death clearly and outcomes of legal verdict may prove to be costly for the entire team of people who performed this operation.

If this was the hurdle of problems for a surgeon and multispecialty hospital due to error in medical record writing, one can imagine what will be the difficulty faced by a dentist who practices independently who may not even possess a written record of the patient details or medical history.

This brings an extreme important of dental record maintenance in clinics with medical history and referral from different specialists duly copied and filed for further reference. All dental specialists must write in a prescription or dental file events leading to any adversity in the dental clinic. This also should also include emergency drugs available, resuscitation apparatus, and O_2 cylinder usage during the adverse event.

By this way the dental specialist will be able to defend his case in court of law if confronted and court of law will be convinced that the dentist had all infrastructure necessary for patient safety in case death or other emergencies.

The following are examples of what is typically included in the dental record:

- Database information, such as name, birth date, address, and contact information
- Place of employment and telephone numbers (home, work, mobile)
- Medical and dental histories, notes and updates (if any referral notes from other doctors)

- Fitness letters from other medical specialists
- Progress and treatment notes
- Conversations about the nature of any proposed treatment, the potential benefits and risks associated with that treatment, any alternatives to the treatment proposed, and the potential risks and benefits of alternative treatment, including no treatment,
- Diagnostic records, including charts and study models
- Medication prescriptions, including types, dose, amount, directions for use and number of refills
- Radiographs
- Treatment plan notes
- Patient complaints and resolutions
- Referral letters from cross consultations.
- Patient noncompliance and missed appointment notes
- Follow-up and periodic visit records
- Postoperative or home instructions (or reference to pamphlets given)
- Consent forms
- Conversations with patients dated and initialled (both in-office and on telephone, even calls received outside the office)
- Correspondence, including dismissal letter; if appropriate

Other information best left out of the record would be personal opinions or criticisms. Stick to facts, especially those related and relevant to providing dental and surgical care. Imagine what you write in a record being read in a court of law (remember that this is a legal document). Do document a patient's refusal to accept the recommended treatment plan and cancelled appointments.

References:

1. Devadiga A. What's the deal with dental records for practicing dentists? Importance in general and forensic dentistry. Journal of forensic dental sciences. 2014 Jan;6(1):9.

2. Surbhi Wadhwani et al. Maintenance of antemortem dental records in private dental clinics: Knowledge, attitude, and practice among the practitioners of Mangalore and surrounding areas. Journal of Forensic Dental Sciences / Volume 9 / Issue 2 / May-August 2017

Autopsy and Forensic Medicine

11.1 Introduction

An autopsy, often referred to as a post-mortem examination, necropsy, or autopsied cadaver, is a highly skilled surgical technique that entails a detailed examination of a body by dissection in order to ascertain the reason and manner of death as well as to assess any possible diseases or injuries. In clinical medicine, autopsies are performed to spot medical mistakes.

Whether it is obvious or damaging to the patient, a medical mistake is an avoidable and unfavourable result of treatment. A misdiagnosis or inadequate treatment of an illness, accident, syndrome, behaviour, infection, or other affliction may fall under this category. According to estimates, 142,000 people worldwide passed away in 2013 as a result of negative medical treatment outcomes, up from 94,000 in 1990.[1] The annual death rate in the U.S. alone was 251,454, according to 2016 research on the number of deaths brought on by medical mistakes, raising the possibility that the 2013 worldwide estimate may not be correct.

According to Prof. Jha's research from Harvard, 5.2 million medical mistakes occur each year in India. Similar to other developing nations, India is not registering many medical errors, according to a report in the British Medical Journal. This is due to a lack of clinical outcome measurement training for physicians and nurses.

Our primary goal is to heal patients; thus, developing a nationwide index of clinical or medical mistakes hasn't been possible for us. The National Accreditation Board for Institutions, established in 2005, is currently gathering information from 350 institutions during the previous five years.

Once this information is gathered, we shall be able to create a national index, ask the other hospitals in the nation to serve as benchmarks, and determine where we stand in relation to other emerging or developed nations. Even in the US, there are 44,000 to 98,000 fatal medical errors per year[2]. Medical mistakes are not the result of a doctor's lack of medical expertise or understanding, but rather of poor teamwork and communication during a crisis. Human error is to blame for almost 70% of deaths brought on by medical malpractice, according to Dr. Rakshay Shetty, a paediatric intensivist at Rainbow Hospitals in Bengaluru, India. In comparison to dental mortality, deaths from medical conditions and treatments are comparatively far more frequent.

On the number of fatalities at dental clinics in India or in other nations, there are no statistics available. The literature does contain erroneous reports of these instances. Every 40,000 dental procedures involving anaesthesia in dental offices result in a reported one mortality. [3] The use of general anaesthesia prior to dental treatment was shown to have resulted in 178 fatalities in England between 1965 and 1999. [4]

An extensive exterior and interior examination of the corpse following an unnatural death is known as a thorough forensic autopsy. In order to help determine the cause and manner of death, the forensic pathologist or medical examiner may, if required, request any tests, additional investigations, and/or consultations with experts anywhere on the globe.

The primary uses of the autopsy are

- Identification or confirmation of the cause and manner of death
- investigation into the nature of the disease and the identification of particular diseases
- advancement of medical practice through the clinical application of autopsy findings

The new uses of the autopsy include

1. Public education,
2. a repository of tissues and organs for transplantation and research,
3. quality assurance of medical diagnoses and services
4. The creation of precise mortality data,
5. The early detection of infectious, environmental, and occupational health risks,
6. Information documentation for upcoming legal, financial, and medical evaluations

7. Evaluation of novel therapeutic approaches and diagnostic techniques;
8. Physicians' on-going education.

11.1.1 Procedure Statement

Fatalities where an autopsy may shed light on unidentified and unexpected medical problems

- Deaths for which the reason cannot be determined with clinical certainty
- Cases where an autopsy may be able to reassure the grieving family, the grieving public, and/or both in regards to the death.
- Patients who have taken part in clinical studies (protocols) that have been authorized by institutional review boards pass away.
- Every obstetric fatality.
- All infant and child fatalities.
- Death at any age if it is believed that an autopsy would reveal a known or suspected condition that might also affect survivors or organ transplant recipients.
- Deaths that are known to have occurred as a result of workplace or environmental dangers
- Sudden, unexpected, or inexplicable hospital fatalities that appear natural and are not beyond the purview of forensic medicine
- Unexpected or inexplicable deaths that occur during or after any diagnostic or therapeutic dental, medical, or surgical treatment
- Natural fatalities that are often covered by forensic jurisdiction, such as those that occur when a patient is hospitalized and those in which the patient appears to have suffered an injury

- Deaths are brought on by infectious illnesses and high-risk infections, such as AIDS. Policies and practices for managing such instances should be agreed upon by pathologists and personnel.
- Patients who have had organ or tissue transplantation and have passed away within 60 days after getting a transplant from a deceased relative.

11.1.2 Autopsy Facts

An autopsy is the process of examining a deceased person's body.

- An autopsy may be limited to a particular organ or bodily part.
- The objective of autopsies is to establish the cause of death. They are often done for legal, educational, and research reasons.
- A service with an open casket is not hampered by the opening of the body.
- Over the previous fifty years, the autopsy rate has decreased from 50% to less than 10%.

11.1.3 How is An Autopsy Performed?

The scope of an autopsy can range from a thorough investigation to a single organ, such as the heart or brain, being examined. Most pathologists undoubtedly see the examination of the chest, abdomen, and brain as the typical scope of the autopsy. Starting with a thorough exterior inspection, the autopsy commences. In addition to recording the body's weight and height, distinguishing features like scars and tattoos are also noted.

A Y- or U-shaped incision from both shoulders connecting across the sternum and going down to the pubic bone is made before the internal examination begins. The rib cage and abdominal cavity are subsequently made visible by separating the skin from the underlying tissues. **(Figure 11.1)**

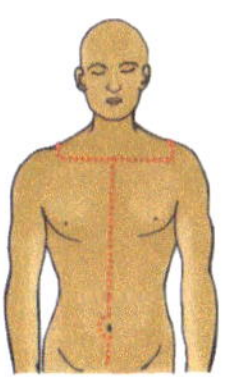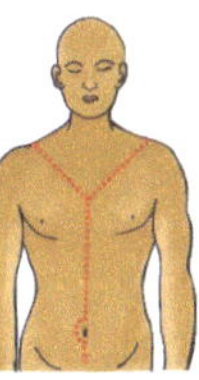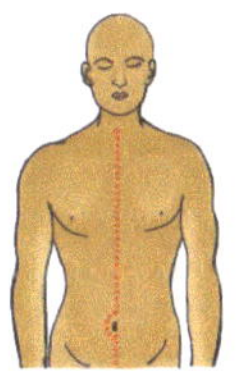

Figure 11.1: Types of Autopsy Incision

To reveal the neck and chest organs, the front of the rib cage is removed. The trachea, thyroid, parathyroid, esophageal, heart, and thoracic aorta can all be removed through this hole. The abdominal organs are separated from the body after the neck and chest organs have been removed. The bile duct system, pancreas, spleen, adrenal glands, kidneys, ureters, urinary bladder, abdominal aorta, and reproductive organs are a few of them.

An incision is made from one ear to the other at the rear of the skull to extract the brain. The scalp is sliced and dragged forward, and the skull underneath it is separated. A vibrating saw is used to remove the top of the skull. After that, the entire brain is carefully removed from the cranial vault. The spinal column's front or posterior half can also be removed in order to access the spinal cord.

The pathologist initially looks over the organs to look for any alterations that are obvious to the naked eye. Atherosclerosis, liver cirrhosis, and coronary artery disease are a few examples of disorders that can cause changes that are easily seen in the organs.

The organs are often taken from the body, separated from one another, and then further dissected to check for any internal abnormalities, such as malignancies. All organs are routinely subjected to small-scale sampling in order to create slide preparations for microscopic inspection. The body's incisions are stitched shut when an autopsy is complete. The organs may be used for education, research, and diagnostic purposes, or they may be kept and returned to the body. As none of the incisions made to carry out the autopsy are visible after the body has been embalmed and dressed by the mortician, doing an autopsy is not disruptive to an open casket burial ceremony.

What other special studies may be done as part of the autopsy?
It is possible to snap pictures of the results for later use. Special studies might involve genetic research, chemical analysis to evaluate medication levels or metabolic problems, or cultures to find infectious pathogens. For upcoming diagnostic or research purposes, tissue might be frozen. Organs can be preserved and kept in formalin for future investigation, sampling for microscopy, conference presentations, or archiving for the instruction of medical students.

What is an autopsy report?
A thorough report that includes a description of the autopsy process, microscopic results, a list of all the diagnoses, and an overview of the case is created when all the tests are finished. The correlation or link between pathologic findings (those derived from the autopsy) and clinical findings (those gleaned from the doctor's examination, lab tests, radiological results, etc.) is highlighted in the report.

What is the percentage of routine autopsies in India?
Government officials are deeply concerned about recent allegations concerning a decline in autopsies because they fear that it could imperil India's sickness and mortality figures. For instance, studies have found that less than 1% of patients who pass away in nursing homes have their bodies autopsied.

Since only 40% of fatalities in India take place at home, it is necessary to utilize an acceptable, low-cost, technology-driven technique to determine the cause of death using verbal autopsy. The development of smartphone applications for the registration of important events may be one feasible answer given the government's vision for a "Digital India" and the extraordinarily quick mobile penetration rate. There are some things that can only be learned during an autopsy. Autopsies can yield information that is useful to society, the medical community, and families. Many medical professionals think autopsies should be reinstated. It remains to be seen if it will be revived.

11.2 Integrating medicine, law, and ethics (autopsy and the law)

"Death is a mystery to the living, and the living look to death for help."

Forensic medicine deals with crimes against people where a medical examination and supporting documentation are necessary. The majority of it involves using common sense in conjunction with information and experience already gained through studying other areas of medicine, dentistry, surgery, etc.

In an ideal world, there is no replacement for fundamental intellect and clinical proficiency. Forensic practice requires a wide variety of theoretical knowledge as well as experience, common sense and an open mind to new options. The forensic pathologist understands that certain results are produced due to biological variation, and there could be an element of uncertainty in many cases. That is why *probability and proof* are two ends of forensic science.

In court, a doctor or dentist should try to earn respect, understanding, and credibility. A doctor should be objective, fair, and truthful. He should be vigilant to hunt for evidence, note everything in detail for a convincing case, and keep in mind that theory and ambiguity have no place in forensic medicine or in evidence presented in court. A doctor is required to tell the whole truth without holding anything back or embellishing. Actually, the doctor does not testify in support of or against the prosecution or defense. Though many extensive forensic medical histories have been explained starting in 1532 in Europe, In India, the history of forensic medicine can be traced back to the Indus Valley civilization, where weapons of various types and users have been depicted. In the Vedas and Samhitas, various symptoms of wound charms, poisoning, and toxicology have been described and well-determined.

An Indian pioneer in this area is Dr. Jaisin P. Modi, who did extensive research in this area while working at Agra and Lucknow medical colleges and published a book that is still considered an authority in this area. The police system of criminal investigation was introduced in India in 1861 and the coroner system in 1871 in the old presidential towns of Calcutta and Bombay.

Due to increasing society needs and significant role in forensic medicine, a medico-legal institute was opened in Bhopal in 1977, and a standing committee on forensic medicine has been established in the Bureau of Police Research and Development under the Ministry of Home Assassins in New Delhi. The Indian Academy of Forensic Medicine was established in 1972.

11.2.1 The Coroner System

A coroner is one of the most ancient systems in the English legal system and one that retains a considerable amount of power. *In India, the coroner system only applies to Bombay and Calcutta at present.* Although the coroner system is present, in practice the system is not in vogue in Calcutta, and the police eventually look after the job. In other Indian states, the report of the inquest is usually done by the **police force** prior to the autopsy.

Cases reportable to the coroner:
According to coroner rules 1953–1980 (consolidated), the following deaths should be reported to the coroner:

1. When the deceased patient has not been treated by the doctor for his last illness
2. When the attending doctor has not seen the patient within 14 days before or after the death.
3. When the demise happened during a procedure or prior to anaesthesia recovery
4. When there is suspicion about the circumstances of a death or when it occurs suddenly while the person is in the dentist chair,
5. When the death might be due to a disease, accident, violence, or any kind of poisoning.
6. Alleged negligent treatment

11.2.2 Legal Procedure for Autopsy

The moment the physician or dentist declares a suspicious death in a dental chair or a dental hospital, an investigation into the cause of death is done. This enquiry by the police force into the cause of death is called an *inquest.*

Police inquest: (S.174, Cr. P.C.)
The police officer in charge will visit the place of offence (a dental clinic, for instance, or a hospital where a dead body was kept) and conduct an inquest in the presence of two or more witnesses. The preparation of a possible cause of death will be judged by the surroundings and appearance of the body. This includes a description of the treatment done, any injuries inflicted, fractures found on the body, bleeding from the mouth or nose, etc.

The success or failure of an investigation depends on the initial observation and actions of police officers at the scene of the offence. These are also responsible for protecting from damage everything that might interest a medico-legal expert.

The visit by the police officer should be as early as possible, and the doctor or dentist will be questioned about
1. Who is the victim? Name, age, sex, etc.
2. Is it your regular patient?
3. Previous dental records, if any, are available?
4. Where and at what time does the death occur: in the chair or waiting hall?
5. Whether the patient has any previous medical history and what medication they used to take
6. Any injuries, bleeding, or asphyxiation occurred?
7. Was any there an external incision obvious outside body?
8. The inquest officer may make a sketch of the direction and position of blood on the body or on the ground.
9. What does the dentist think about death, and how did it happen?
10. Whether the death is unnatural or inflicted due to surgery or negligence
11. Whether the patient had medical fitness or if he or she was receiving care from other specialists who were treating patients
12. Have any attempts been made to rescue the patient from the death or drugs administered?
13. What drugs have been administered in dental clinics?
14. Was there any known allergy?
15. Was there any negligence in drug administration, drug dosage, etc.?
16. Was proper consent taken for high-risk surgeries in the clinic?
17. Did he inform immediately the duty medical superintendent or medical director in charge of the hospital if death occurred in a hospital setting?

Coroner's inquest: It is held only in Bombay.

Magistrate's inquest: It is done by an executive magistrate in cases of (a) death in prison (b) while in police custody (c) due to police firing (d) exhumation (S.176Cr P.C.). This is especially crucial if family members allege foul play in connection with dental treatment complications following a death, and subsequent complaints can only be heard if a magistrate holds an inquest in place of or in addition to the police inquiry.

11.2.3 Preservation of Medico-legal Evidence

Evidence must be gathered legally from the scene of the death, be pertinent to the case, and be approved by qualified specialists before it can be used in court.

1. It is of paramount importance that at the scene of death, all material evidence regarding a case will have to be protected by the dentist for the defence, labelled specimens of an argument. This may require complete notes, medical records, photographs, drugs, x-rays, gloves, syringes, and forceps that must be correctly labelled and marked.

2. Do not alter anything of medico-legal value. Do not cut, alter, or tear clothing or crucial evidence.

3. Store and transport specimens as necessary in clean containers.

4. Do not try to tamper with evidence or records, as they may be counterproductive defense-labeled specimens.

5. The scene may be examined by an evidence specialist for marks on the body, CPCR signs, ecchymosis, etc.

6. If any foreign body from the throat is retrieved, present it for examination (like a denture, reamer, etc.).

All deaths in a dental clinic or hospital should be treated as unnatural unless proved otherwise. Things may not always appear right at first sight. But on thorough investigation, a negligent or accidental death may be more evident from records, evidence, and the circumstances of the issue. Many times, even a small suspicion of foul play warrants an autopsy, as the history given by the patient or relative cannot be relied upon.

It is the duty of the police inquest officer to decide whether an autopsy is necessary or not. The dentist or surgeon cannot deny to proceed with autopsy, if asked by the police. In the same way, they cannot insist on an autopsy if relatives are not willing to undergo it for the body.

11.2.4 Why is Autopsy Mandatory in Medico-legal Cases?

The ultimate problem faced by the criminal justice system the world over is identifying the cause of death. The forensic science comes to the task of solving these known and unknown mysteries, and the medico-legal fact of death is thus said process after various tests is known as `autopsy`. (post-mortem examination)

The literal meaning of the word autopsy is 'itself-examination' which does not signify anything particular, particularly the fact of getting data from a dead body. Experts feel better terminology would have been necropsy, meaning `an examination of the dead`.

There are four types of autopsies:

1. Clinical autopsy:
When the examination confirms the diagnosis of the causes of death and the cause of death is known or frequently believed to be known in error. The main goals of this are educational, instructive, and research-related.

2. Medico-legal autopsy
A medico-legal autopsy is an examination performed under the law for the protection of its citizens. The function of a medico-legal autopsy is to find some or all of the following facts:

1. To find the cause of death
2. To identify the body

3. To find out whether the death is natural or unnatural
4. To find out the time of death
5. Presence of poisons or chemicals in the body
6. Nature and number of injuries
7. To allow proper recovery and preservation of evidence
8. To provide a correlation of facts and circumstances related to the death

Medical aspects of death:

For insurance purposes, one must consider the following:

a) the anticipated length of life;
b) the presence of natural disease and its contribution to death, which also includes trauma;
c) the interpretation of injuries caused by criminal, suicidal, accidental, or negligence; and
d) the analysis of the death for and related to surgical or medical procedures.

3. Verbal Autopsy (VA)

A verbal autopsy relies on an interview with the deceased's relatives or other close friends to determine the cause of death. A structured questionnaire is used throughout the interview to obtain details on warning signs, symptoms, medical history, and events leading up to death.

Based on the information gathered using the VA questionnaire and any additional information that may be available, the cause of death or the series of reasons that resulted in death are determined. In order to identify the cause of death, the VA questionnaire may be used in conjunction with rules and regulations, algorithms, or computer programs. The components of a typical VA instrument include a VA questionnaire, a list of causes of death or a mortality categorization system, and sets of diagnostic criteria (either expert or algorithmic algorithms derived from data) for determining causes of death. The cause-specific mortality fractions that are determined through the VA method depend on a variety of parameters and go through a number of processes.

Due to the lack of vital data from the Civil Registration System, the Office of the Registrar General of India has adopted an alternate strategy to have lay reporters in rural regions and medical attendants in urban areas record the reasons for death on a sample basis. These reports are sent to the State Vital Statistics Office by the Municipal Health Office in urban areas and the primary health centers (PHCs) in rural regions.

4. Social Autopsy

A social autopsy is a thorough examination of a wide range of psychosocial factors underlying fatalities that affect a specific group of individuals. However, verbal autopsy data can be used to rank health issues and assess the effectiveness of health programs. Social autopsy data, which focuses on modifiable factors present in the home, community, and health system, may guide policies and practices for increasing access to and utilization of preventive and curative services. The information provided by social autopsy, for instance, can raise awareness that maternal and infant mortality are avoidable, enable communities to actively engage in measures to lower these numbers, and improve the responsiveness and accountability of health programs.[2]

Remember an autopsy will tell only the cause of death and who caused it (the person himself like self-injury or other). But it cannot pinpoint who did the crime, so it is only corroborating evidence to prove the guilt of the person.

11.3 **Format for Crime Scene**

(Modifiable-keep it simple and handy, it can be plain paper also)

Ref. Letter ……………………   Telephonically called………………

PM …………………………   No ………………………………

Date ……………………………   Time ………………………………

Time of arrival to scene …………………………………………

Location …………………………………………………………

Weather condition at scene ……………………………………

Temperature ……………………   Humidity level ……………………

Outside weather at Morgue ………………………………………

Accompanied by …………………………………………………

Investigating Officer of case ……………………………………

Initial Information / PCR Record

Observation of surrounding

Observation of victim
- Position
- Clothing
- Wounds

Time since Death
- Decomposition,
- Rigor Mortis,
- Post-Mortem Staining
- Core body temperature
- Apparent injuries
- Any other significant findings
- Insects
- Blood / stains spatter
- Items found in vicinity
- Sketches
- Impression (lip / bite marks)
- Any advisory to IO (Inquest Officer) and his team
- Camera used

Signature

Key points in the autopsy:

Inquest papers required for conducting a postmortem

1. Post-mortem request: a must
2. Any medical or legal certificate is preferred.
3. Police Form 25/35A, B, or C, depending on the situation:
4. Seizure Memo (Products Seized at Scene): Desirable
5. CSI team evaluation of the crime scene and photos—prefer (The full scene may be downloaded onto a CD or flash device.) Overall scenario information is particularly beneficial since, without it, medical personnel and investigators would waste valuable time on conjecture and guesswork.
6. Statements from the public, the sarpanch, or family are preferred.
7. An account of the patient's treatment and death at the hospital would be ideal.

An autopsy will only be performed if a police officer, coroner, or magistrate issues a formal written order. If an inquest report is not provided, a doctor cannot decline an autopsy. In the same manner, a doctor is not required by law to perform autopsies on anyone who is presented to him.

- Autopsy should be performed in a mortuary in daylight as soon as possible and should never be performed in private rooms. It must be remembered that advanced purification is difficult to transport, may lose evidence, and should be conducted in a local, available mortuary without delay.
- No relatives, politicians, or lawyers will be allowed inside during the autopsy, apart from the in-charge police personnel.

- Identification, photographs, and marks should be clearly mentioned and noted.
- A forensic pathologist to corroborate the cause of death can read the inquest report and do an examination on the basis of direct evidence.
- The doctor will be able to go through the case records provided by the specialist surgeon or dentist.
  - The forensic specialist can show the police officer any additional injury if it is not mentioned in the inquest, and necessary corrections can be made.
  - If there is a special risk involved with a deceased person, like AIDS, the autopsy must be done in a specialized mortuary meant for the same.

In a similar vein, the doctor should refrain from doing an autopsy if the dead individual happens to be a close family member or friend.

The Autopsy Protocol

A protocol is a written record that has been signed and is used to prove anything.

Two types of autopsy records will be written: *Numerical: using figures; narrative: using stories*

Once the deceased individual has been delivered to the mortuary, the date, time, and police-produced evidence will all be recorded in the mortuary register.

A complete autopsy will involve the examination of three great cavities in the body, and the organs contained in them (all cavities) should be carefully examined, even though an apparent death of cause is found in one of them. It is better that an autopsy is done by an experienced hand in cases of medico-legal issues, as many things may be missed if a junior-level pathologist examines without having enough experience. The dentist will have no say in suggesting who should do an autopsy.

11.4 Stages in Postmortem Examination

After the body is received by the doctor, the examination is done in two stages:

11.4.1 External Examination

The following are observed:
- Description of the dead body: age, colour, and weight
- Description of the extremities
- Evidence of a fracture, old or recent
- A detailed description of wearing apparel and marks
- Body length, height, and complexion
- Scalp, tattoo marks, condition of the eye, teeth
- Discharge from the mouth and nose
- Potation or biting of the tongue is noted.
- Haemorrhage, if any external
- Any blood stains, mud stains, etc. noted
- State and distribution of rigor mortis noted
- Cadaveric spasm
- State of decomposition noted
- Presence of maggots or other insects
- Adipocere, or mummification of the body
- Ligature marks or sutures in the body
- External injuries

It is possible to compare exterior and interior damage using photographs. X-ray examination can be used to locate any radiopaque objects or instruments, deformities, or plates from surgical procedures, swallowing, or aspiration. The external examination will try to find out the probable cause of death, including what type of injury and weapon may have caused death and struggling marks in cases of homicidal nature.

11.4.2 Internal Examination

The three different body cavities are to be opened in a planned way.

Incisions:
A midline incision that runs straight down from the chin to the symphysis pubis and passes either to the left or right of the umbilicus marks the beginning of an internal examination.

The cranial cavity is opened with two incisions. The examination of neck structures requires three different incisions. Some prefer to open the chest cavity first, and others open the abdomen first.

Abdomen: After examining the external wall of the abdomen, the recti muscle is slit open; the contents are cut at separate levels and examined for the condition of the cavity and the relationship of organs to one another. The contents will be examined for inflammation, strain, hemorrhagic points, ulceration, and the smell, color and character of the substances. The splanchnic vessels may be examined for thrombi or emboli. Also, the examination of fluid, pus, or any other foreign material like dentures, endodontic files, and gauze should be done. The color of the organs, the weight, and the consistency of the organs will be checked.

The liver, spleen, pancreas, kidneys, adrenals, bladder, and prostate are examined separately for any additional findings apart from the already-mentioned assessment.

Neck: Through the platysma of the upper jaw, the neck is dissected laterally to the side of the neck, and all the contents are from one another. The dissection will follow from submandibular to tongue, palate, and prevertebral muscles. The neck structures are grasped in one mass and pulled down to chest level. The tongue should be examined for bite marks, the presence of bruises, etc. The carotid should be examined for thrombosis, and the tracheal pharyngeal area should be checked for the presence of blood, vomited matter, and foreign bodies.

The chest: The chest is cut open through rib cartilage and examined for blood, foreign bodies like prosthetic dentures, files or reamers, orthodontic brackets, or any other dental surgical implants or instruments that may have been accidentally slipped into the lungs, resulting in mortality. If pneumothorax is suspected after a major road traffic accident, it must be examined for fluid and air and noted separately. The lungs and pulmonary vessels should be examined for emboli if there is a suspected death from pulmonary embolism.

Heart: The heart is examined morphologically in each area, including the great vessels, pulmonary artery, valves for thrombosis, stenosis, infarction, and plaque formation.

Head: After extending the neck with wooden blocks under the shoulders, a coronal scalp opening (intermastoidal incision) is done from behind the ear to the opposite side. The skullcap is removed and the brain is examined for extradural or intradural haemorrhage or any areas of stroke or infarction.

The ear, spine, genitalia, and extremities are examined separately.

Unless they are needed for additional research or to be used as evidence in a future trial, all organs that have been taken from the body shall be given to the deceased person with their appropriate locations for burial.

The dissected parts are brought together and well sutured after washing the entire body.

Specimen Collection

Preservation of autopsy parts in medico-legal cases like death in dental practice where the cause is not known

Apart from routine autopsy, the following structures must be preserved for further investigations if police request the doctor to preserve the viscera if foul play is suspected in the death of the patient:

Specimens like blood, urine, bile, vitreous humor, CSF, stomach contents, and loops of small and large bowel will be collected during the postmortem. The ideal sample for DNA profiling is blood. When blood is not a possibility in degraded situations, teeth are the next best sample.

The autopsy surgeon should sample from the following list:

1. Femoral blood collection
2. Vitreous humor aspiration
3. CSF aspiration
4. Synovial fluid collection from the knee, elbow, and ankle
5. Stomach content collection
6. Blood collection from the heart
7. Collection of material for culture: blood, pus, and cavity fluids
8. Blood-soaked, dried gauze piece
9. Smear preparation
10. Swabs from different parts of sexual assault, bite marks, foreign material, etc.
11. Material for DNA profiling: blood, bone, muscles, teeth

12. Extracting and preserving teeth
13. Cutting and preserving long bones
14. Rub fetal skin with your fingertips.
15. Scrape nails
16. Trim nails
17. Comb pubic hair
18. Pulling and clipping pubic hair
19. Collection of head hair (pulling and clipping)
20. Plant material on the skin and in clothes
21. Soot and combustible debris from clothes, ears, and nostrils
22. Preparation of a blood smear
23. Aspiration of sphenoid sinus fluid
24. Body surface swabs
25. Samples of histology taken from various organs
26. Diatom sampling in drowning cases
27. Gunpowder residue swabs in weapon instances, paraffin cast preparation
28. Collecting tissue, blood, and stains on the scene or from moving vehicles, etc.
29. Urine should not be less than 100 ml, either via catheterization or through a transdermal needle and syringe aspiration.
30. Liver: to study toxicity

The tissue parts being investigated are preserved either in a saturated sodium chloride solution or rectified spirit. Normally, the tissues are not preserved in formaldehyde because many chemicals from the tissue make it difficult.

Separate, clean bottles should be used for small parts of the viscera, blood, and urine, and the bottles should be well labelled and fitted with glass stoppers. The preservative should be in equal volume to the tissue content; otherwise, the bottle might burst due to decomposition and gas formation. The bottle head should be sealed and labelled with the date, name, part mentioned, and place of biopsy. The tissue parts sent for examination should also include a copy of the inquest and postmortem report. [1]

11.5 Negative Autopsy

Even after thorough study, it is occasionally challenging to ascertain the cause of death in forensic situations.

- Before declaring the case a negative or obscure autopsy, proper screening through medical history, histopathology of the vital organs, toxicological screening, crime scene evaluation, drug interaction, envenomation, hypersensitivity reaction due to new protein material, vaso-vagal inhibition, concealed injection, and air embolism must be done.
- Negative autopsies can also be caused by insufficient training, insufficient and inappropriate external and internal inspection, incomplete medical examination, and failure to attempt histopathology and toxicological analysis.

The following guidelines are recommended if a negative autopsy is declared:

1. Evaluate the scene and record all relevant medical history, including palpitations, syncope, dizziness, snoring, the posture in which the deceased were discovered, the ventilation in the room, sexual asphyxia, mental disease, substance abuse, etc.
2. Inspect clothing and check pockets for any drugs or abuse materials, including suicide notes.

3. Full-body photography with a close-up

4. Perform a thorough examination of the body to look for any concealed injections or injuries.

5. Before beginning the autopsy, samples of the vitreous, blood, and urine are taken for toxicological testing, and blood smears are made to check for haematological abnormalities such as anaemia, leukaemia, pancytopenia, etc.

6. Checking fingers and palms for hazardous substances

7. Check the oral cavity and any samples taken for harmful substances.

8. Check the respiratory track, oro-pharynx, larynx, and mouth for any bolus or aspiration.

9. Check for an air embolism.

References:

1. Abubakar II, Tillmann T, Banerjee A. Global, regional, and national age-sex specific all-cause and cause-specific mortality for 240 causes of death, 1990-2013: a systematic analysis for the Global Burden of Disease Study 2013. Lancet. 2015 Jan 10;385(9963):117-71.

2. Lebanon N, Hanover N. How many deaths are due to medical error? Getting the number right. Eff Clin Pract. 2000;6:277-83.

3. O.P. Murty et al. Uniform guidelines for postmortem work in india: Faculty development on standard operative Procedures (sop) in forensic medicine and toxicology. Journal of Forensic Medicine & Toxicology Vol. 30 No. 1 & 2, January - December 2013

4. Kalter HD, Mohan P, Mishra A, Gaonkar N, Biswas AB, Balakrishnan S, et al., et al. Maternal death inquiry and response in India - the impact of contextual factors on defining an optimal model to help meet critical maternal health policy objectives. *Health Res Policy Syst* 2011; 9: 41- doi: 10.1186/1478-4505-9-41pmid: 22128848. (Social Autopsy)

Forensic Dentistry – An Overview

Forensic Odontology is a branch of forensic sciences that involves evaluation of dental evidence in crime scene investigation. It has all the more important role when the dental remains are the only available evidence as in cases of extremely decomposed or mutilated bodies as in floods and aviation disasters. Knowledge in this field is fast growing with technological advancement. This chapter offers an overview and covers collectively various aspects of forensic odontology under following broad topics

• Dental Records
• Teeth and jaws
• Radiographic aspects
• Histological aspects
• Molecular methods

12.1 Dental Records

Importance of maintenance of dental records play a vital role in individual identification more so in mass disasters like earthquakes, cyclones, train and aviation accidents, wars and terrorist activities. Maintaining records can be in the form of dental charts, casts, radiographs and photographs. Dental chart should be detailed with information such as name, gender, age, address, occupation, dental and medical history, details of the teeth present, missing and filled teeth, dentures, variations in the morphology of teeth and mucosa with supportive photographs and radiographs. In India, dental records should be mandatorily maintained and retained for at least 3 years from the commencement of treatment. For children the records are expected to be preserved up to 25 years of their age. Orthodontic models pre and post are to be retained permanently. During mass disasters, disaster victim register (DVR) with yellow coloured ante-mortem forms and pink-coloured post-mortem forms are processed into electronic version called DVI (Disaster Victim identification) system International. In India, clear guidelines, quality assurance programs are the need of the hour more so for private practitioners.

12.1.1 Age Estimation Based on Eruption of Teeth

Based on the eruption pattern and status of teeth in the oral cavity, estimation of age is considered to be one of the simplest and reliable techniques. Based on the chronology charts, the age of the individual will be identified.

12.1.2 Chronology of Teeth Eruption

Primary Teeth	Central Incisor	Lateral Incisor	Canine	First Molar	Second Molar
Maxilla (In Months)	8 – 12	9 – 13	16 – 22	13 – 19	25 – 33
Mandible (In Months)	6 – 10	10 – 16	17 – 23	14 – 18	23 – 31

Permanent Teeth	Central Incisor	Lateral Incisor	Canine	First Premolar	Second Premolar	First Molar	Second Molar	Third Molar
Maxilla (In Years)	7 – 8	8-9	11– 12	10 – 11	10 – 12	6 – 7	12– 13	17– 21
Mandible (In Years)	6 – 7	7 – 8	9 – 10	10 – 12	11 – 12	6 – 7	11– 13	17– 21

12.1.3 Personal Identification Based on Tooth Morphological Features.

Certain morphological features of teeth aid in individual identification. Additionally, habits in certain occupations bring about alterations in morphology of teeth. Forensic dental comparison also includes the comparison of the dental fillings, surface structure / root configuration, crowding of teeth, spacing in between the teeth including diastemas, teeth rotations, transpositions, any supernumerary teeth, developmental disturbances, type of occlusion etc.

Morphological features used in individual identification	
Hard Tissues Central Incisors	Shovelling Hutchison Incisors / Diastema / Mesiodens Flattened/ Wedge Shaped abrasion in between incisors (In Tailors – Biting needles / sewing thread) Nail marks in the incisors (In Electricians / Cobblers / Nail biters) Mesiodens Pink intrinsic discoloured teeth indicative of Strangulation, Suffocation or drowning
Lateral Incisors	Peg Laterals (Microdontia)
Canines	Minor distal groove Talon Cusp
Premolars	Dens Invaginatus Dens Evaginatus
Molars	Carabelli's Cusp / Hypocone / Protostylid / Paramolar / Distomolar / Mulberry Molars / Anodontia (3rd Molars)

Morphological features used in individual identification	
Bite Mark	They are documented based on size, location and severity. Helps in differentiating attack injuries and defensive injuries. Tooth pressure marks, tongue pressure marks and tooth scrape marks are documented for analysis. Based on arch shape, teeth size, pattern of injury and location, bite mark of humans and animals are differentiated.
Soft Tissues Cheiloscopy	Identification of a person based on various patterns like vertical, branched, intersected and reticulate types.
Rugoscopy	Rugae are asymmetric, irregular ridges on the mucous membrane of the palate. Their uniqueness to every individual aids in person identification based on shapes like pointed, straight, curved, angled, sinuous, circular, Greek, calyx shaped, racket-shaped and branched types.

12.1.4 Gender Determination Based on Tooth Dimensions.

Certain teeth exhibit variations in dimensions between males & females and this sexual dimorphism can aid in gender determination. Of all the teeth, mandibular canine dimensions exhibit significant difference between males and females. Mandibular canine Index (MCI) helps in gender prediction with an accuracy of about 75-85%. MCI is calculated using the mesio-distal measurement of canine and intercanine arch width. Males have greater MCI in comparison to females.

12.1.5 Gender Identification Based on Cranio-facial Features

Dimensions and the morphology of the craniofacial complex contribute to sex differentiation. Morphology of the skull as well mandible along with a constellation of six other traits (mastoid, supraorbital ridge, size and architecture of skull, zygomatic extensions, nasal aperture, and mandible gonial angle) are used in gender identification. Age estimation using this technique shows accuracy upto 94%. Studies have proved sex differentiation using frontal sinus (mucosa lined air spaces situated between the internal and external laminae of frontal bone) measurements in which the width, height and area of the frontal sinus were found to be greater in males with distinctive difference in shape, measurements, and symmetry.

12.1.6 Differences in Skull Morphology Between Males and Females

Features	Male	Female
Constellation of six traits		
Size and architecture of skull	Larger and Rugged	Smaller and Smooth
Supraorbital margin	Round	Sharp
Mastoid	Medium – Large	Large – Medium
Zygomatic Bone	More pronounced	Less pronounced
Temporal Ridge	More Prominent	Less Prominent
Mandible Gonial Angle	Less obtuse	More obtuse
Frontal sinus dimensions		
Length, Width and Area of Frontal Sinus	Larger Increases with age, decreases after the age of 45 Years	Smaller Increases with age, even after 45 years
Other possible craniofacial features		
Superciliary Arch	Large and pronounced	Small
Nasal Aperture	High, thin, sharp margins	Low, wide, rounded margins
Mandible	Squared	Rounded
Teeth Size	Large	Small
Inter-canine Distance	Greater	Lesser

12.2 Radiographic Methods

Dental radiographic techniques such as OPG, CT scan, MRI and IOPA play an important role in the registration, collection, detection and preservation of forensic evidence in relation to oral cavity. These records are non-destructive and add significance during comparative dental identification using ante and post mortem radiographs in age/gender estimation and reconstructive identification. For identification of victims where putative identity remains unknown, radiographs play a major role in reconstruction. It is always not necessary to have ante-mortem radiographs to identify the individual. Hand written dental records of the individuals obtained from clinics can be used to compare with the post-mortem radiographs. Especially in burns cases, where there is unavailability of tissues for DNA analysis, radiographs play a vital role particularly if the person has any developmental anomaly, making the identification easier.

Fractures in cranio-facial region can be identified whether they are peri or post mortem and also, the time of extraction can be assessed based on the extraction sockets in the radiographs. Any calcification present in the soft tissues like calculi in the salivary gland ducts, tonsils and bullets in gunshot injuries can also be detected based on their distinct opaque appearance.

Radiographic evidence is confirmatory evidence and without radiographic evidence, the individuals age, sex and other pertinent details are not accepted in the legal forums.

Unlike in the past, with recent technical advancements, it is now possible to make radiographs in the crime scene itself with equipment like transportable scanners that have become cheaper and post mortem dental scans are performed in a short duration of time. Scanners help in assessing areas that are difficult to access thereby focusing autopsy on particular region or in some instances eliminating the necessity of autopsy.

12.2.1 Utility of Radiographs in Age Estimation

Radiographically, the mineralization of deciduous incisors is seen at the 16th week of intrauterine (IU) life. Before the mineralization of tooth germs, they appear as radiolucent areas on the radiograph. A radiograph of the mandible taken at the 26th week of IU life shows advanced mineralization in anterior teeth with 3/5 th crown completion at the 30th week of IU life. In the newly born fetus, completely fused cusps for the deciduous first and second molars are seen whereas there is evidence of tip of one of the mesial cusps alone within the crypt of the permanent first molar.

Age estimation: description based on radiographs	
Schour and Masseler method	Describes 21 chronological steps from 4 months to 21 years of age, and, developmental charts were published. Calcification stages of teeth on radiographs are compared with the standards.
Moorees, Fanning and Hunt method	Based on 14 stages of mineralization in development of single and multi-rooted permanent teeth, age correlation was done in comparison to the corresponding stage of development. Development of teeth in female was notably ahead in comparison to males.
Demirjian, Goldstein and Tanner method	Tooth mineralization of seven mandibular permanent teeth from second molar (M_2) to central incisor (I_1) was determined and graded into eight stages (A to H). The obtained score will be converted directly into a dental age as per the standard table given or by using regression formula. Separate formula for males and females have been mentioned.
Nolla's method	Mineralization of permanent teeth has been evaluated in ten stages. Comparison between radiographs and pictorial representation has been provided for age assessment. Separate table of age estimation for males and females are given with and without involvement of third molar.

Age estimation: description based on radiographs

Kvaal's method	This method is used to estimate age in adults and is based on assessment of volume of teeth. Pulp tooth ratio will be evaluated for six teeth of maxilla and mandible using which age will be estimated. Measurements considered in Kvaal's technique are maximum tooth length, maximum pulp length, maximum root length on mesial surface on cemento enamel junction to root apex, root and pulp width at cemento-enamel junction, mid point between cemento-enamel junction and mid root length and at mid root length.
Coronal Pulp cavity Index	This method is used to estimate age in adults using the fact that coronal pulp cavity reduces as the age increases due to secondary dentin deposition. Pulp was calculated using panoramic X-ray photographs. Parameters considered are height of the crown and height of the pulp cavity.
Harris and Nortje method	This method is based on the third molar root development. Five stages of 3rd molar development is correlated with age. Five stages includes I – <1/2 root length; II – ½ root length; III- 2/3/ root length; IV – wide open apical foramen; V – closed apical foramen
Van Heerden system	Development of mesial root of third molar was correlated with age using panoramic X-rays.
Cameriere method	Age estimation is calculated by ratio between length of the projection of open apexto the entire length of tooth major axis. Left seven permanent mandibular molars are used. Standardized for both single root and multi-rooted teeth.

12.3 Histological Aspects in Forensic Dentistry

The hard structural component of the teeth namely enamel, dentin and cementum are histologically different and have characteristic histologic features to adapt to the various mechanical and physiological challenges encountered during growth and development. It has been established those certain histological aspects like incremental lines of retzius, neonatal line (in enamel), von ebner lines, secondary dentin, dentin translucency (in dentin), salter's incremental lines (in cementum) aid in age estimation and these structures thereby play an important role in anthropological studies and in investigating alleged stillbirths in female infanticide cases.

12.3.1 Enamel

Prism cross striations and Incremental lines of Retzius

Ameloblasts which secrete enamel proteins follow a circadial rhythm in their metabolic activity at regular intervals of nearly 3-4um which is close to a 24 hour cycle representing daily variation in rate of secretion and mineralization in enamel prisms and are called prism cross striations. Mean of 7-8 cross striations between two striae of retzius indicate close to weekly periodicity of the retzius lines. For any individual, the number of prism cross striations inbetween striae of retzius remains constant for all teeth. Total cross striations counts are consistent with those expected from the known age and thereby the period of survival of infant can be estimated from the total number of cross striations from the established neonatal line (**Figure 12.1**).

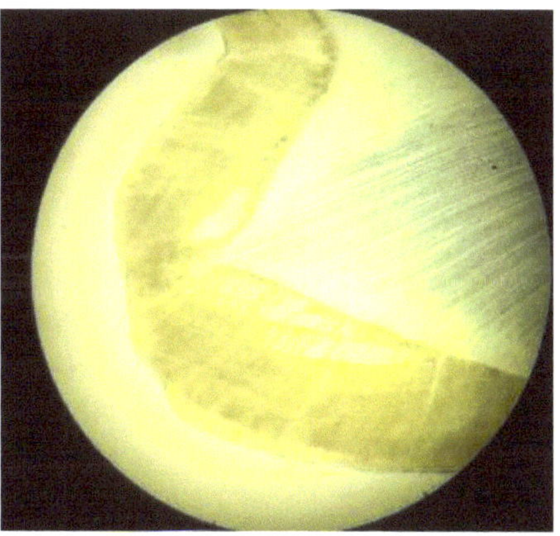

Figure 12.1: Incremental lines of Retzius

Total number of perikymata ranges from 130-190. Changes in number and size of these wave like markings have been noticed in modern humans in comparison to hominins (**Figure 12.2**).

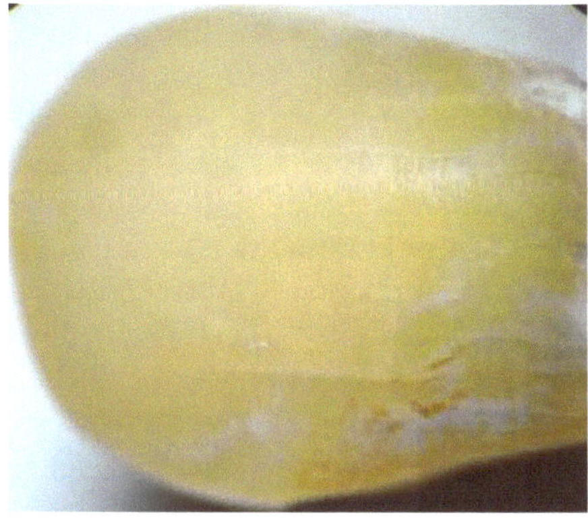

Figure 12.2: Perikymata

12.3.2 Enamel Rod and Patterns

Perikymata - Macroscopic enamel rod end patterns

Wave like markings on the outer surface of the teeth-enamel are called as perikymata. Macroscopically, Enamel rod formation in incremental pattern is manifested as perikymata on the tooth surface They have depth varying from 2-5 um with spatial periodicity ranging from 50-100um. These are the external manifestations of the incremental lines of Retzius and appear as linear grooves. Each perikymata takes upto 6-12 days to form in modern humans. These linear grooves are highly susceptible to physical and chemical damages. Perikymata reflects duration and speed of crown formation thereby playing a major role in palaeoanthropology to classify and identify fossils. They also provide insight into dental development in human fossils compared to modern human samples.

12.3.3 Tooth Prints – Microscopic Enamel Rod End Patterns

Microscopically, enamel rod ends run in various directions and form patterns called tooth prints which are considered as alternatives for finger biometrics. In an individual, each tooth exhibits distinct tooth print and the study of these tooth prints are called as Ameloglyphics.

12.3.4 Neonatal Line

It is an accentuated incremental line, 12μm in width, which delineates enamel formed before and after birth. It is seen only in deciduous teeth and in mesio-buccal cusps of the first permanent molars and is absent in rest of the permanent teeth. Presence or absence of neonatal lines can aid in investigating alleged still births in cases of female infanticide.

12.3.5 Dentin - Incremental Lines

Dentin is deposited with daily incremental pattern of 6μm in crown and 3.5μm in the root and the cyclic activity of odontoblast in 24 hours is manifested as lines of Von Ebner. These fine striations are perpendicular to the dentinal tubules and are about 4-8mm apart in crown and appears closer in root. The accentuated incremental lines are called lines of Owen. These lines indicate disturbances in matrix formation and are areas of hypomineralization. Neo natal line delineates dentin formed before and after birth thereby aiding in investigations of female infanticide.

12.3.6 Root Dentin Translucency

Root dentin translucency, both in terms of length and area, increases with age thereby aiding in age estimation by taking single rooted ground sections into observation. This region is least affected by environmental factors and the pathological processes. As the age advances the translucency progresses in the coronal direction. Estimation of age using area of dentin translucency showed good association with original age in comparison to age estimated by comparing the length. Length and area of the dentin transparency is calculated using manual or digital methods. And the recorded parameters are analysed using regression statistical analysis. With increase in age by one year the length of the dentin translucency increases by 0.77 mm and area of translucency increases by 0.80 mm².

12.3.7 Secondary Dentin

The band of dentin that is surrounding the pulp and formed after the root completion is secondary dentin. Its formation is a slow and continuous process and its deposition is more prominent at the roof and floor of the pulp. Secondary dentin is usually assessed in three areas coronal 1/3rd, middle 1/3rd and apical 1/3rd in a ground sectioned tooth under microscope and average thickness of the secondary dentin is calculated. Secondary dentin can be used in conjunction with other parameters or it can be used as sole parameter in regression equations to estimate the age **(Figure 12. 3)**.

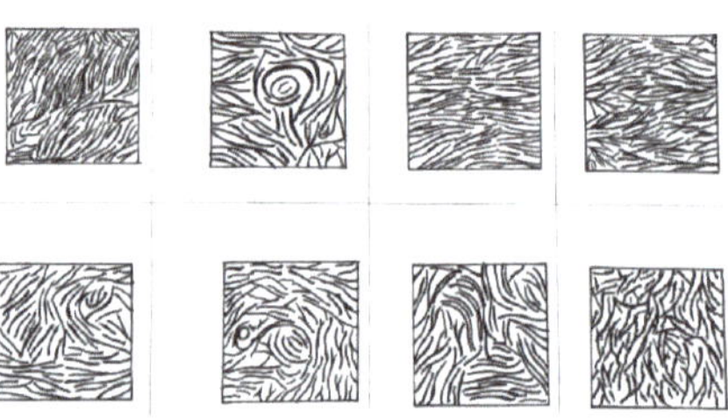

Figure 12. 3: Tooth Prints

12.3.8 Cementum

Tooth cemental annulation (Figure 12.4)

Cementum has the property of continuous apposition throughout the lifetime thereby forming incremental lines. This augmented apposition is caused due to relative variation in mineralization and collagen orientation. Areas of rapid tissue growth appears as light bands and areas of reduced tissue growth appears as dark bands. A pair of light and dark bands represents one incremental line. Usually it takes a year for one increment line to appea Based on these incremental lines age can be estimated using the formula

Estimated age = Eruption age of tooth + Total width of the cementum / width of the cementum between two incremental lines.

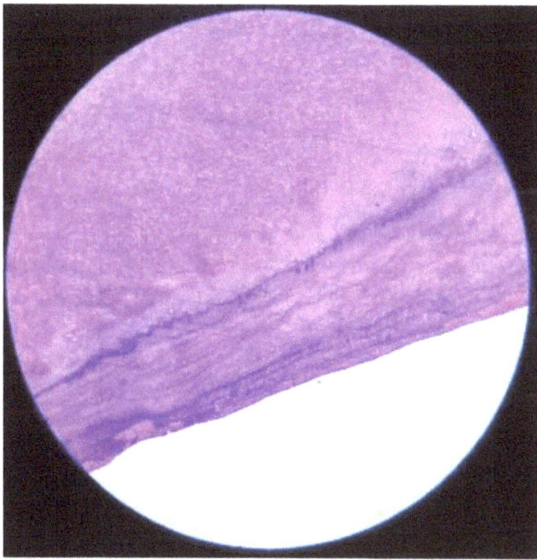

Figure 12. 4: Tooth Cemental Annulations

12.3.9 Gustafson Method

In Gustafson's method (1950) teeth are used for age estimation, taking into consideration six parameters such as root resorption, translucency, cementum apposition, secondary dentin, periodontosis and attrition. The ground section of teeth are evaluated microscopically and all the variables are scored from 0-3 based on the severity and age is calculated using the regression formula

Estimated age = 11.43X+(4.56* X)
[X- total score]

Mean error calculated in Gustafson's index is +/- 3.6 years. Later, many modifications were proposed to the Gustafson's method. Gustafson/Johanson modification is the most accepted method of age determination.

12.3.10 Amino acid Racemization

Amino acid racemization is a technique by which age of an individual is estimated using the age dependent non enzymatic changes in amino acids (L-form to D-form) that occurs in enamel/dentin/cementum. Dentin aspartic acid racemization is highly reliable in comparison to enamel or cementum. Amino acids during their formative stages are usually in L form and during their lifetime some are converted into D-form due to racemization. Based upon the racemization rate, the age of an individual is estimated. Racemization process is highly sensitive to temperature and pH, thereby cooling of body after death affects the process. In tooth specimens of post-mortem age above 20 years, age cannot be estimated effectively by this method. Alternatively, enamel can be used for the study as it is more resistant to environmental changes but the level of proteins is low and this challenges their isolation and age estimation.

12.3.11 Barr bodies

Barr and Bertram in 1949 identified a small chromatin condensation in neural cells of female cats. Barr body is a small, well defined, darkly stained body present in nuclei of cells of female origin and are absent in male cells thereby helping in gender identification. It represents condensed inactive X chromosome (heterochromatin). These bodies are also evident in bone cells, retinal cells as well oral mucosal cells. Studies suggest that Barr bodies can be studied histopathologically from tooth pulp tissue at various temperatures thereby aiding in gender identification in mutilated and charred bodies where pulp is encased and protected by the surrounding hard tissue structures.

12.4 Molecular Methods

12.4.1 DNA Profiling

The role of DNA profiling in victim identification has its roots from 1985. From the identification of micro satellites to gender determination by genomic dot blot hybridisation DNA profiling from dental hard tissues serve as the last hope of person identification in various crime scene investigation and mass disaster victim identification. Dentin and pulp serve as a source of DNA in a tooth. Genomic DNA and mitochondrial DNA are two types of DNA that could be extracted from a tooth. Various techniques that have been employed in identification of genomic material and effective DNA fingerprinting are restriction fragment length polymorphism, polymerase chain reaction, short tandem repeat typing and of recent micro array techniques and next generation sequencing. DNA offers a huge clearance in many crime investigations. Teeth can withstand extreme temperature changes and DNA from cells of various structures of the tooth (pulp and odontoblastic processes) are shielded as they are encased by hard tissue thereby contributing as effective source of DNA.

12.4.2 Mitochondrial DNA

Mitochondrial DNA (mtDNA) is special in forensic investigations due to its exclusive maternal inheritance. The mitochondria of the sperm are eliminated from the cytoplasm of the oocyte after fertilization by specific nuclease dependent systems, autophagy and ubiquitin proteasome system. Also, as these mitochondria in the sperm are present in the tail and are lost during fertilization. Therefore, paternal mitochondrial DNA is never transmitted to the offspring, thereby mitochondrial DNA aids in tracing maternal lineage in forensic investigations. Isolation and profiling of mtDNA is a very technique sensitive process. Recent advances in DNA profiling have eased the procedure.

References

1. Nanci A. Enamel: composition, formation and structure. In Ten cate's Oral Histology Development, structure and function, 141-190, Mosby Elsevier, 2008

2. Sivapathasundharam B, Adaptation editor. Shafers Textbook of Oral pathology. 9th ed. India: Elsevier; 2021.

3. Smith TM. Experimental determination of the periodicity of incremental features in enamel. J Anat. 208(1): 99-113, 2006

4. Antoine D, Hillson S and Dean MC. The developmental clock of dental enamel. a test for the periodicity of prism crossstriations in modern humans and an evaluation of most likely sources of error in histological studies of this kind. J. Anat. 214: 45-55, 2009

5. Skinner M and Anderson GS. Individualization and enamel histology: a case report in forensic anthropology. J Forensic Sci 36: 939-948, 1991

6. Skinner M and Dupras T. Variation in Birth timing and location of the

neonatal Line in human enamel. J Forensic Sci 38(6): 1383-90, 1993

7. Ramenzoni LL and Line SRP. Automated biometrics-based personal identification of the Hunter-Schreger bands of dental enamel. Praoc R Soc B 273:1155-1158, 2006

8. Ohtani S and Yamamoto T. Strategy for the estimation of chronological age using the aspartic acid racemisation method with special reference to coefficient of correlation between D/L ratios and ages. J Forensic Sci 50:1020-7, 2005

9. Griffin RC, Moody H, Penkman KEH and Collins MJ. The application of amino acid racemization in the acid soluble portion of enamel to the estimation of the age of human teeth. Forensic Sci Int 175:11-16, 2008

10. Slavkin HC. Sex, enamel and forensic dentistry: A search for identity. J Am Dent Assoc 128: 1021-25, 1997

11. Sweet D, DiZinno J A. Personal identification through dental evidence-tooth fragments to DNA. J Calif Dent Assoc 1996; 24: 35-42.

12. Pretty IA, Sweet D. A look at forensic dentistry–Part 1: The role of teeth in the determination of human identity. British dental journal. 2001 Apr;190(7):359-66.

13. Weedn V W. Postmortem identifications of remains. Clin Lab Med 1998; 18: 115-137.

14. Dorion R B. Disasters big and small. J Can Dent Assoc 1990; 56: 593-598. 8. Malkowski F S. Forensic dentistry, a study of personal identification. Dent Stud 1972; 51: 42-44.

15. Brannon R B, Kessler H P. Problems in mass disaster dental identification: a retrospective review. J Forensic Sci 1999; 44: 123-127.

16. Clark D H. An analysis of the value of forensic odontology in ten mass disasters. Int Dent J 1994; 44: 241-250. 1

17. Solheim T. A new method for dental age estimation in adults. Forensic Sci Int 1993; 59: 137-147.

18. Shapiro H L. Forensic anthropology. Ann N Y Acad Sci 1978; 318: 3-9.

19. Whittaker D K, Rawle L W. The effect of conditions of putrefaction on species determination in human and animal teeth. Forensic Sci Int 1987; 35: 209-212.

20. Chandrashekar C, Takahashi M, Miyakawa G. Enamel and Forensic odontology - Revealing the identity. Journal of hard tissue biology. 2010;19(1):1-4.

21. Sweet D, Hildebrand D, Phillips D. Identification of a skeleton using DNA from teeth and a PAP smear. J Forensic Sci 1999; 44: 630-633.

22. Hongwei S, Jingtao J, Cameron J M. Age determination of the molars. Med Sci Law 1991; 31: 65-68.

23. Ogino T, Ogino H, Nagy B. Application of aspartic acid racemization to forensic odontology: post mortem designation of age at death. Forensic Sci Int 1985; 29: 259-267.

24. Liversidge H M, Molleson T I. Developing permanent tooth length as an estimate of age. J Forensic Sci 1999; 44: 917-920.

25. Nunn J, Shaw L, Smith A. Tooth wear-dental erosion. Br Dent J 1996; 180: 349-352.

How to Break Bad News: A Guide for Clinicians

CHAPTER
13

Any information that negatively and significantly influences a person's perception of their future is considered to be bad news; nevertheless, one's perception of what constitutes bad news is subjective.

There are several circumstances that require the practicing dentist and maxillofacial surgeon to inform patients and their loved ones of terrible news. Breaking terrible news without the correct training can have detrimental effects on patients, families, and doctors themselves.

Unfortunately, dentists and maxillofacial surgeons have hardly had any training in this aspect during their undergraduate or postgraduate programs. Delivering bad news is a difficult task for all. Breaking terrible news puts our communication abilities to the test. These discussions may be quite delicate for both the doctor and the patient. It makes a big difference when the correct things are spoken in the appropriate ways. Many experts may have just briefly known their patients while they were inpatients or outpatients.

Poor communication has been linked to negative clinical and psychosocial outcomes, including decreased pain tolerance, non-compliance with treatment, misquoting or misunderstanding prognosis, and dissatisfaction at not being involved in decision-making. This is especially true for cancer patients and patients who have experienced trauma. Patients who have passed away while receiving dental care also exhibit this.

For the clinician, poor communication results in a lack of job satisfaction, increased stress, and a high percentage of mistakes and complaints. The physician has to be able to understand the patient's emotions and respond appropriately as they deal with the trauma that receiving bad news causes, in addition to their verbal communication skills.

Possible reactions of people who are suddenly bereaved [1]

The medical staff should be ready to handle a wide variety of emotional outbursts since reactions to the news of a sudden death are frequently strong. The way that individuals react to untimely death is influenced by their cultural, socioeconomic, and ethnic backgrounds. People may weep while wailing, shrieking, or making loud, exaggerated gestures with their bodies. Each person experiences grief differently, and it might differ from one person to the next. The grieving family members may exhibit the following mourning emotions because they feel that the abrupt loss was "untimely" and "unfair."

- Initial shock reaction.
- Denial: After receiving unexpected and distressing news, denial is a typical phenomenon that should

be acknowledged and allowed. Encourage family members to visit the corpse of the deceased, especially those who were not present when the person passed away or was in danger of passing away, to help them come to terms with the loss.

- Anger: This depends on the incident's specific circumstances. Many people find it difficult to accept the death of a close friend or relative. In India, aggressive conduct is fairly typical. Physicians, hospital employees, and occasionally hospital property and equipment may display this. After being aired, anger will eventually subside.
- Guilt: Guilt is the internal manifestation of resentment and self-blame. The medical staff's comforting comments will aid in overcoming this feeling.

There are rules that may be followed to enhance successful communication and prevent unpleasant situations. The recommendations made in this chapter are meant to serve as straightforward advice for doctors and should not be taken as official protocols. The framework created by Baile and Buckman (2000) is one that health professionals find useful. The elements highlight the key ideas to keep in mind while informing patients and/or their loved ones of terrible news. These may change depending on the situation, the gravity of the news, the parties involved, the amount of planning time, etc.

"In general, however, the better the outcome is likely to be, the more detailed attention that can be given to each of these factors. preparing the speech, paying attention to the audience, and seeing their various reactions. The atmosphere must be treated with the utmost care, and discussions and the conduct of the medical staff will have a significant impact on the patient and family in every way.

Here, an extensive, step-by-step modified action plan for delivering the bad news and easing grief is offered.

The SPIKES protocol is a set of six steps for breaking bad news.

(S- Setting, P- Perception,
I- Invitation or Information.
K- Knowledge, E- Empathy,
S- Summarize or Strategize)

Step 1: Setting Up the Interview
The goal should be to provide the ideal physical environment, prioritize privacy, minimize interruptions, assist patients in understanding and listening, uphold confidentiality, and offer support. If required, contact will be facilitated by having affiliated doctors and paramedical professionals present. The doctor must put the patient at ease and reassure them after gathering all pertinent data and test findings.

The following points must be taken into consideration:

1. Quiet and private counselling room for confidentiality
2. Deciding who should break the news
3. How many doctors and staff should be present
4. Planning how to start conversations
5. Hospital staff must sit at the same level as the patient or relative.

STEP 2: Assessing the patient's perception

It is important to find out how much the patient or relative knows about the events during the hospital stay or about the debilitating medical issues the patient is suffering from. The following points must be clearly understood for a healthy discussion.

- Is there awareness among relatives regarding the past medical issues of the patient?
- Updates given by the doctors or hospital staff regarding earlier admission
- Emotional content of the patient's response
- Words and physical gestures of the doctor and patients' relatives This may indicate a level of anxiety between the parties.

Step 3: Obtaining the patient's invitation

In any discussion concerning terrible news, find out how much the patient wants to know. Not "do you want to know?" but rather "at what level do you want to know?" is the true question. This might be a contentious topic.

Informed decisions and consent: Knowing how much the patient or their loved ones want to know specifics will help when providing information about the current course of therapy. Clearly a leading question, "You don't want to be bothered with the details, do you?"

The physician must be dedicated to giving the patient accurate and thorough information.

Questions are worded in this direction, depending on the context. "Would you like me to tell you the details of the diagnosis?" is one example of a question. Are you the type of person who prefers to be fully informed if this turns out to be anything serious?

Step 4: Giving the patient knowledge and information.

- Make a decision first about your interview goals.
- Our objective shouldn't leave us unprepared.
- Don't disregard the patient's comments.
- Do not obfuscate the truth in order to further your goals.
- The diagnosis, treatment strategy, prognosis, and support may need to be explained to relatives.
- Family members are free to accept or reject our explanations and decide whether to continue therapy as necessary. Additionally, people are free to express their opinions however they see fit.
- Reiterating essential facts is crucial because people who are angry or surprised find it difficult to understand or recall specifics.
- Use textual messages and diagrams as tools. Utilize memoirs, audiotapes, or pamphlets; pay attention to the questions or responses that are provided "between the lines".
- Invite patients to ask inquiries. Be prepared for cross-questioning. When a worried party requests clarification, there shouldn't be a break in the conversation.

Step 5: Addressing the patient's emotions

Breaking unpleasant news is a challenging challenge. Responses from the patient might range from muteness to sorrow, denial, or wrath. Pay attention and be patient with the affected. Ask them how they are feeling or thinking as you acknowledge their loss. Some people might not want to continue listening and show this through their emotions or body language. As requested, permit stillness. In addition to being willing to listen to them, we must also be emphatic and empathetic.

Empathy enables the sufferer to communicate their emotions and concerns while still feeling overwhelmed. Allow emotional expression without judgement and avoid conflict.

Step 6: Strategy and summary planning
Demonstrate professionalism and compassion throughout the interview. Explain to them about hospital support and other sources of help, if necessary. Each session will help us improve and effectively tackle patients and relatives in a sensitive manner. All personnel, including doctors and hospital staff, should be taken on board in the sensitization of issues and instructed to maintain a unified explanation. Every communication must be entered in the patient's records for future reference to help face any untoward medical-legal issues arising in the future.

Ideal action plan:
- In the event of an event, initiate communication by informing appropriate persons.
- Privacy and confidentiality are to be maintained.
- A senior member should lead the discussion.
- Be prepared with all documents from the time of admission until the event.

- If mortality happens in a dental chair or clinic premises, explain how quickly you responded to resuscitate or move the patient to the hospital.
- Explain, with clarity, the possible reason for morbidity or mortality.
- Allow the relatives to go through the grief and give them time.
- If the patients' family criticize or condemns the medical staff, hospital, or dentistry clinic, do not engage or quarrel with them.

Medical students and physicians should be taught the art of communication, just as pilots do with simulators. Like any other facet of medical care, this ability has to be taught. This will help us generate doctors or dentists who are better prepared to handle this challenging but crucial area of clinical medicine.

References:

1. Naik SB. Death in the hospital: Breaking the bad news to the bereaved family. Indian journal of critical care medicine: peer-reviewed, official publication of Indian Society of Critical Care Medicine. 2013 May;17(3):178.
2. Baile, W. F. (2000). SPIKES—A Six-Step Protocol for Delivering Bad News: Application to the Patient with Cancer. The Oncologist, 5(4), 302–311. doi:10.1634/theoncologist.5-4-30.
3. Baile WF, Buckman R, Schapira L, Parker PA. Breaking bad news: more than just guidelines. J Clin Oncol. 2006 Jul 1;24(19):3217.

Medical / Dental Negligence in India - An Overview

14.1   Introduction

Medical negligence has numerous meanings. In the infamous case of Blyth v. Birmingham Waterworks Company (1856), Baron Anderson defined negligence as "the doing of something that a prudent and reasonable man would not do, or the omission of doing something that a reasonable man, guided upon those considerations which ordinarily regulate the conduct of human affairs, would do." If the defendants accidentally performed something that a prudent person would not have done or failed to do something that a prudent person would have done, they may have been negligent. The term reasonable' is the key word in the definition. This establishes the bar for judging the "standard of care," whose failure is the core of carelessness. [1]

We comprehend that the following elements must exist in order for a behaviour to be deemed negligent:

- A specific level of care was required of the doctor.
- The physician did not uphold that standard
- That the carelessness caused harm (the damage should be covered by insurance).
- The irresponsible act and the harm it caused should be closely related.

In actuality, all four of the aforementioned requirements must be met for an act to qualify as medical negligence. One must wrestle with the negligence exclusions in order to comprehend negligence. An examination of court-decided instances reveals that certain of the below-listed circumstances do not constitute medical negligence. Examples include not obtaining informed permission in an emergency situation, patient unhappiness with the course of therapy, and even charging exorbitant amounts. [2]

Important considerations in negligence: A level of care or expertise that is established by a body of experts on behalf of the medical profession is typically referred to as the professional standard of care. This does not have to be done with the utmost care. 'Reasonable care' is used in this situation. The "Bolam test" has long been used to evaluate standards [3]. The Bolam Test allows for two or more divergent viewpoints in the management of a certain ailment and is used to assess the scientific validity of a claim. Two crucial features of therapy or care must also be taken into consideration in this situation.

They are:
1.   Customary practice
2.   Accepted practice

A frequent practice might be a custom. However, it is not recognized by law if it is not supported by science. Contrarily, established practice is typically founded on facts and is recognized by legislation. For instance, many individuals forego using rubber dams during root canal therapy. Although that could be common practice, it is incorrect. However, even if rubber dams are not always utilized, using them is a recognized practice. Only the established procedure will be followed in the event of an accidently ingesting an instrument.

A mitigating circumstance in the culpability for carelessness is contributory negligence. The defendant doctor may argue that there was no carelessness on their part if the patient helped lead to a negative outcome. For instance, a patient may not have taken a medicine as directed.

14.2 Liability for negligence

A doctor, dentist, or hospital accused of negligence may be held accountable under one of three categories. When a doctor's actions fell below the standard of reasonable care, rather than when the patient really was hurt, that is when the doctor becomes liable. In other words, a doctor is not always responsible for the harm that a patient experiences. Only those that are a result of a duty breach make him accountable.

The risk might be
1.   Civil liability (torts)
2.   Criminal liability
3.   Statutory liability

Due to the inclusion of medical services within the Consumer Protection Act (1986), there are still additional obligations in India. This occurred as a result of a protracted legal dispute in IMA (Indian Medical Association) v. VP Shantha and others, which ultimately decided that medical service was categorically included in the definition of service contemplated under the Consumer Protection Act, which is a quasi-judicial legal presumption intended to provide prompt justice in the event of a deficiency of service. Typically, civil or tort responsibility applies.

If found guilty of civil culpability, the defendant must pay the complaint unliquidated damages that may be either simple or exemplary, depending on the judge's (or a jury's, in many countries) decision.

Negligence in some circumstances may result in criminal penalties, such as jail time, fines, or both. In India, however, there are cases that have been determined, such as Jacob Mathew v. State of Punjab 2005, where rigorous criteria have been established for criminal action against physicians. They cannot be detained unless a medical board rules that the negligent act was truly criminal in character and resulted in death or impairment during treatment. Provisions 337, 338, and 304A (rash and negligent act causing simple damage, grave injury, or death, respectively) of the Indian Penal Code are pertinent provisions.

There are statutory organizations in several nations, including India, that have the authority to launch investigations into negligent actions by medical and dental practitioners who are registered with those organizations. They may impose sanctions ranging from license suspension to requiring retraining prior to returning to practice. [3,4]

Medical negligence is something that physicians and dentists need to be aware of in order to take the proper precautions and avoid needless legal action.

References:

1. http://en.wikipedia.org/wiki/Blyth_v_Birmingham_Waterworks_Company/
2. Paul G. Medical law for the dental surgeon. Jaypee; 2004.
3. Bolam Vs Friern Hospital managing committee. (1957) 2 AIIER 118
4. Rao SJ. Medical negligence liability under the consumer protection act: A review of judicial perspective. Indian journal of urology: Journal of the Urological Society of India. 2009 Jul;25(3):361.
5. Pandit MS, Pandit S. Medical negligence: Coverage of the profession, duties, ethics, case law, and enlightened defense - A legal perspective. Indian J Urol. 2009 Jul;25(3):372-8. doi: 10.4103/0970-1591.56206.
6. Ji YD, Peacock ZS, Resnick CM. Characteristics of National Malpractice Claims in Oral and Maxillofacial Surgery. J Oral Maxillofac Surg. 2020 Aug;78(8):1314-1318. doi: 10.1016/j.joms.2020.03.015.
7. IMA v VP Shantha and Oths 111 (1995) CPJ

Medical and Death Audit

An audit of clinical practice is the analysis of data either prospectively or retrospectively to determine both quantitatively and qualitatively the work load of an institution or individual department. It includes numbers of admissions, patient demographics, various complications and mortality.

Medical audit is a planned program with an objective of monitoring and evaluating all aspects of dealings in medical care of all practitioners in a hospital or a department which then identifies areas for improvement through a mechanism of action taken, corrected and sustained those improvements for future optimal clinical care.

Surgical audit is a normal part of surgical practice. It is a systematic, critical analysis of the quality of surgical care provided, with the aims of improving quality of care, continuing education for surgeons, and guiding appropriate use of health resources. It has certain advantages, e.g. accuracy of data collection, opportunities for clinical learning and training needs analysis, clinical outcome indicators, development of surgical protocols, measures of operational effectiveness, opportunities to identify and correct problems and guidelines for research

Death Audit means a technique or process of quantitative death record analysis & compiling the information pertaining to the professional activities of the hospital, as well as the qualitative analysis & evaluation of the data so collected.

Objectives of Medical Audit:

- The primary purpose of such an audit is to elevate the quality & efficiency of medical care, & for so doing, to seek the cause for poor results
- To improve clinical staffs and administrative personals medico legal safety
- To maintain data/ medical record quality
- Protect current and future funding
- To improve quality of the medical service
- Useful for optimal clinical improvement
- Encourages teamwork
- To improves patient care in wards, theatres and ICUs.
- Financial benefits
- Contractually an obligation as per government policy
- It doesn't involve experiments or research
- For effective utilisation of staffs and facilities available
- Help in developing explicit standards and protocols for treatments.

Objectives of Death Audit include-

- To ascertain the proportion of patients who died because of problems in care.
- To pin point the incorrect treatment or management in specific death on the systems and process.
- To ascertain the team members, the concern / adverse event caused by medical negligence leading to different causes of death.

The medical and death audit in dental and maxillofacial field are very rarely conducted in India in authors knowledge. This is purely due to reasons of very rare occurrence of death within the dental institutions as 99% of the cases done in dental institutions are on an out-patient basis with minimal risk involved. But any invasive dental / maxillofacial specialties can have death in practice though it is sporadic all over India. A medical audit in a dental institution can be performed within specific departments like oral and maxillofacial surgery and pediatric dentistry because of involvement of sedation and general anesthesia. Since most of the major maxillofacial procedures happens within general hospital attached to dental institution / within the premises of medical college campus having dental services facility. Though sporadic death can occur in dental chair as well as medical hospitals attached to dental institutions or private maxillofacial practice, a medical and death audit can be performed to analyze, ascertain and for corrective measures as a team to identify the lacunae and deficiencies of service provided to the population.

LEVELS OF AUDIT

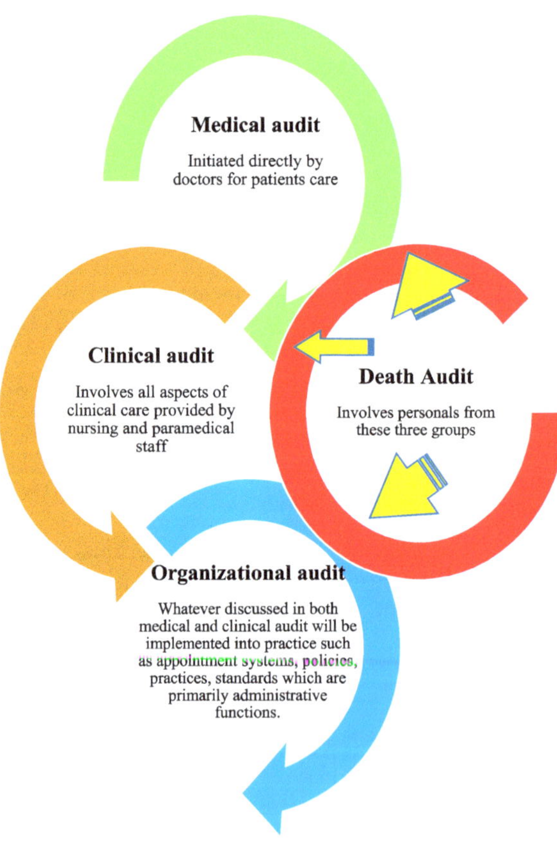

TYPES OF CLINICAL AUDIT

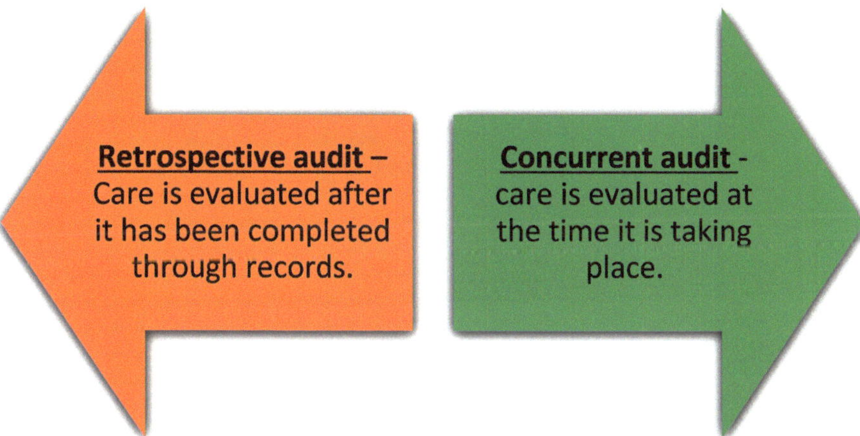

Team:

A team is chosen in medical and death auditing to audit the records. The members must be experienced physicians who judge frank, fearless and without prejudices.

The Team involves - a Forensic Expert, a Pathologist, the Doctor who was in charge of the patient, representative from supportive paramedical department and management team during his or her treatment. Medical accounting or quantitative case record analysis will be done by a trained medical record librarian, in the absence of such a person an intern or a house surgeon should supervise & guide the staff to carry out the analysis.

Steps in medical death audit to improve quality health care:

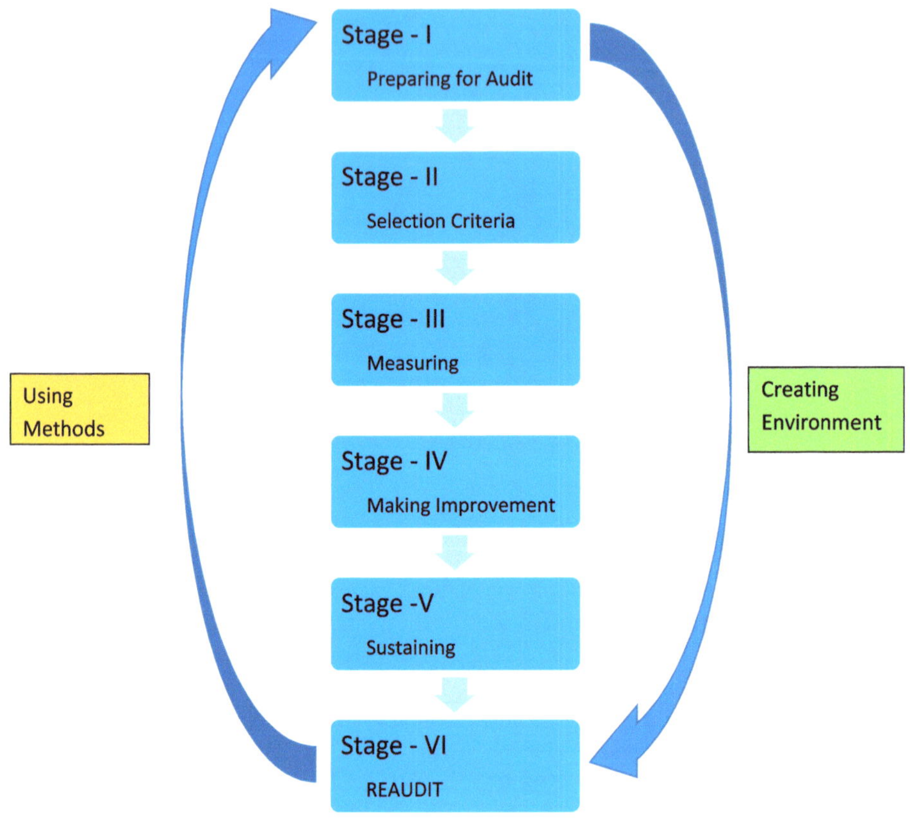

The sample format given below is taken from SAST (Suvarna Arogya Suraksha Trust, India) regarding death audit explaning different levels of inclusion of management of a patient in clinic or hospital setup prior to death.

DEATH AUDIT REPORT

Section A: General Information_________________

Patient details:
Name:
Age: Sex: Pre-auth No.
DOA: Date of Surgery: DOD:
Diagnosis: ____
____

Treatment given: Surgery/Procedure/ Radiotherapy/ Chemotherapy/ Others (specify)
____
____

Hospital name: ____
Name of Treating Doctor: ___________________________________

Section B. Case summary
____

Please provide a summary of the Case in the form of narrative – **including complaints at the time of admission, chronology of events up to death of the patient**

Section C: Case

Assessment____

a) **Were there any areas of CONCERN or ADVERSE EVENTS in the management of this patient?**   Yes   No

b) **Was surgery performed?**   Yes   No

c) **Were there any Areas of Concern, or Adverse Events in any of the following areas if an operation/procedure was performed or treatment provided?**

Discussion points	Yes	No	N/A
Pre anesthetic checkup/fitness for surgery/treatment			
Decision to operate			
Choice of operation			
Timing of operation (too late, too soon, wrong time of day)			
Intra-operative process			
Problems in functioning of OT			
Grade / experience of surgeon deciding			
Grade / experience of surgeon operating			
Post operative period			

a.   Was this patient treated in a critical care unit (ICU or HDU) during this admission?
Yes   No

b.   If no, should this patient have been provided critical care in ICU/HDU?
Yes   No

____

____

Opinion of the Audit committee regarding overall risk of death

Minimal   ☐
Mild   ☐
Moderate   ☐
Severe   ☐

If there any areas of CONCERN or ADVERSE EVENTS in the management of this patient:

1.   Describe the significant event/s during the course of treatment in the hospital:

Note any areas of:

Concern ____

Adverse Event ____

Note if these areas caused any of the following:

Made no difference to outcome ____

May have contributed to death____

Caused   death   of   patient   who   would   otherwise   be   expected   to survive____________________________

Was the death preventable?

Definitely   ☐
Probably   ☐
Probably not   ☐
Definitely not   ☐
Don't know   ☐

____

Section D. Investigations done and their reports

SL NO	INVESTIGATION	REPORT	REMARKS
1			
2			
3			
4			
5			
6			
7			

Section D. Record of cause of death
Hospital mortality audit committee review findings:

Primary cause of death: ____

ICD code: ____

Secondary cause of death: ____

ICD Code: ____

Antecedent cause of death: ____

ICD code: ____

Attestation by the Mortality Audit Committee members:

SL NO	NAME	DESIGNATION	SIGNATURE
1			
2			
3			
4			
5			
6			

Date:

Preparation for Medical and Death Audit:
1. Criteria Development - Admission, hospital services recommended, range of length of stay & indications for discharge, & complications or cause of death.
2. Selection of Cases with Diagnosis
3. Post Mortem report statement regarding the cause of death
4. Worksheet preparation
5. Case evaluation
6. Tabulation of evaluation
7. Presentation of reports

FINAL RECOMMENDATIONS (if any) OF THE MORTALITY AUDIT COMMITTEE

1. ____

2. ____

3. ____

Medical and Death Audit in Dental / Oral and Maxillofacial surgery:

A death from dental / maxillofacial cause it will be a serious concern for the practitioners. Due to the unique anatomical region constituting head and neck & airway, the morbidity and mortality can happen during surgeries, clinical practice which need to be audited.

A precise reflection of data of maxillofacial morbidity and mortality may not reflect a true number as many deaths may be concomitant with other disease of body region including cardiovascular, neurosurgical, casualty and co-morbid medical conditions.

Oral and Maxillofacial Surgery is specialty with an extremely low mortality rate. Respiratory complications are the most common cause of death in patients who survive from maxillofacial trauma. General anesthesia poses a negligible mortality risk to ASA class I patients in comparison to that of an ASA class III and IV patient.

Recommendations based on safe dental and maxillofacial practice to avoid morbidity and mortality in India.

Always there will be basic question which lingers in dentists and surgeons mind that why healthy people have unexplained cardiac deaths and die... There is no definite answer for the same but guidelines help in minimizing complications leading to mortality

1. All patients of maxillofacial trauma or otherwise should be thoroughly examined for any respiratory and cardiac abnormalities and prompt referral must be done from other specialist concerned as when required prior to definitive maxillofacial surgery.
2. The position of any time emergency medicine specialist should be mandatory in all maxillofacial

units that exist outside of a medical hospital.

3. Another study of the same kind should be repeated after every 5 years as a form of a clinical audit to see any improvements or otherwise in the management of patients at this unit.

4. An annual mortality and morbidity conference should be held in the department involving maxillofacial surgeons and allied specialists from the medical field to conduct a critical appraisal of the multidisciplinary treatment approach of patients and suggest ways to decrease the existing morbidity and mortality rate.

5. Residents of Oral and Maxillofacial Surgery should have a minimum of 2 months rotations in a medical or surgical ICU at par with other mandatory rotations fulfilling the requirements for FCPS/MDS.

6. Factors like use of Halothane anaesthetic agent (ventricular arrhythmias) can be avoided.

7. If sedation or GA performed it must be with full monitoring equipment in the form of an ECG, pulse oximeter, non-invasive arterial pressure and a capnograph together with defibrillator should be available; along with fully equipped recovery facility with adequately trained staff.

8. Use of newer inhalational anaesthetic agents like sevoflurane should be implemented in theatres to reduce intraoperative arrhythmias.

9. Appropriate use of airway management devices like fibreoptic bronchoscope is mandatory in all difficult airway conditions.

10. Check list of all instruments used, gauze, throat pack usage, cautery earthing systems and drug dosage must be strictly implemented

---

References:

1. O.P. Murty et al. Uniform guidelines for postmortem work in India: faculty development on standard operative Procedures (sop) in forensic medicine and toxicology. Journal of Forensic Medicine & Toxicology Vol. 30 No. 1 & 2, January - December 2013

2. Islam MA, Haider IA, Uzzaman MH, Tymur FR, Ali MS. One year audit of in patient department of oral and maxillofacial surgery, Dhaka Dental College Hospital. Journal of maxillofacial and oral surgery. 2016 Jun;15:229-35.

3. Basheer Rehman et al. Two years audit of maxillofacial surgery department at Khyber college of dentistry, Peshawar. Pakistan Oral & Dental Journal Vol 29, No. 1, (June 2009)

4. Somnath Das et al. Medical Audit and Death Audit. J Indian Acad Forensic Med, 32(4)

5. Manal Guirguis-Younger et al. Carrying out a social autopsy of deaths of persons who are homeless. Evaluation and Program Planning 29 (2006) 44–54

Negligence Anecdotes

Negligence Anecdotes-1
(Death)
(Criminal Negligence)

A 23-year-old young man with a complaint of mandibular prognathism consulted an orthodontist for treatment of his deformity. He was advised orthodontic treatment followed by surgery. The orthodontic treatment was initiated at a dental clinic under the care of a qualified consultant for a period of 18 months prior to the proposed surgical intervention. Based on joint consultations with an oral and maxillofacial surgeon, the patient was scheduled for surgery in a hospital in town A. The patient, who was an information technology professional in another state, came as instructed for admission to the designated hospital on the morning of surgery.

His pre-op assessment was performed earlier by the anaesthetist, and it was not deemed necessary for the patient to be admitted on the previous day as he had no anticipated risks or co-morbidity (ASA1). The patient was placed on nil per oral and was scheduled for surgery at 9 a.m. He was induced and intubated by a senior anaesthetist and prepared for the procedure. The oral and maxillofacial surgeon, assisted by the dental surgeon under whom the patient was admitted, scrubbed in for the procedure. Soon after the patient was painted with antiseptic preparation, positioned, and draped, the oral surgeon administered 1 ml of 2% lignocaine with adrenaline after due aspiration. Prior to the incision, the anaesthetist stopped the surgeon for an observed change in the cardiac rate and rhythm. Shortly thereafter, the patient was arrested and successfully resuscitated. It was decided by the anaesthetist that the patient should be shifted to a higher centre in view of anticipated hypoxia and serious cardiac deterioration. The patient was arrested again in the ambulance en route and could not be resuscitated.

The body was handed over to the police in view of it being an incident and was sent for an autopsy or postmortem.

All documents and case sheets were seized from the hospital based on a criminal complaint lodged by the parents and relatives.

Allegation of parents and relatives
1. Negligence by doctors
2. Inadequate facility in the operating theatre.
3. Inadequately trained personnel.
4. The parents did not know about the surgery. They only thought that some wires were going to be changed.

Defendants
1. Hospital
2. Dental surgeon and orthodontist
3. Oral and maxillofacial surgeons
4. Anaesthetist
5. Referring dentist

Liability

1. Criminal negligence under Section 304A
2. Civil case under the Consumer Protection Act with the State Consumer Redressal Forum (pecuniary jurisdiction over Rs. 20 lakhs)
3. Statutory complaints with the State Dental and Medical Council

As it stands, the medical board was constituted as per Supreme Court directives. No negligence was found. They were unable to determine the inciting cause. Cardio-pulmonary arrest was the proximate cause of death. The appeal yielded no further information.

Presently being heard by an apex medical board specially constituted under the government (on further appeal by the plaintiff),

Anecdote: 2

Death in the outpatient department

A patient with difficulty swallowing and mild dyspnea following a toothache reported to a dental clinic in town A. He was seen by a dental surgeon and an oral and maxillofacial surgeon. A tentative diagnosis of Ludwig's angina / facial space infection of odontogenic origin was made. It was decided that the patient would benefit from an incision and drainage. The patient was shifted to a small nursing home run by an ENT surgeon. It was decided that there was no need to take the patient to the theatre as it was a septic case, and an incision and drainage were planned in a treatment room that had no monitors or oxygen. As soon as the ENT surgeon administered a IV sedation, the patient stopped breathing and could not be resuscitated. The patient was declared dead after unsuccessful resuscitation with cardiac compression and ventilation with an Ambu bag.

Following public unrest and violence outside the hospital, the patient's body was handed over to the police. This situation usually mandates an autopsy. Eventually, the situation was settled by paying compensation as demanded by the relatives. No criminal, civil, or statutory action was initiated.

Anecdote 3

A middle-aged patient with a space infection secondary to a dental cause reported to the emergency room and was admitted by an oral and maxillofacial surgeon in a teaching hospital. A routine blood investigation showed that the patient was an uncontrolled diabetic. In view of the significant dyspnea and dysphasia, it was decided to perform an emergency incision and drainage under local anesthesia. The assistant professor made the decision to do the procedure in the room adjoining the ward. During the procedure, the patient had a cardiac arrest or respiratory arrest. No monitoring or resuscitation equipment was available, and the patient succumbed. The hospital RMO refused to sign the death certificate as it was not his admission. The head of department refused to sign the declaration of death and refused permission for the assistant professor to sign a declaration of death. The patient's relatives abused and physically assaulted the surgeon, as there was a delay in releasing the body. The police finally arrived to defuse the situation and took possession of the body after a medical officer signed a declaration of death. No postmortem was done as the relatives chose to accept it as a natural death.

An autopsy revealed that the patient had a myocardial infarction. It was entered as a hospital death, and no case was registered. However, several questions on the reason for "no declaration of death" by the attending surgeon were raised, and the matter was unresolved due to the uncertainty of whether the maxillofacial surgeon could have or should have declared death prior to handing over the body to the police. This would have avoided public outrage.

Anecdote 4

A child with dental problems was seen by a pediatric dentist. As the child was not cooperative, it was decided by the dentist and the parents that it would be best to treat the child under general anesthesia / inhalational anaesthesia. The child was scheduled for the procedure at the clinic. An anaesthetist with 'experience' in outpatient daycare surgery was called in to administer anesthesia. He came in with limited equipment and a possible monitoring device. After administering an I/V drug (later believed to be ketamine), the dentist began his procedure with the child under anticipated dissociative anesthesia. The anaesthetist departed with his equipment shortly thereafter. Subsequently, the child developed what appeared to be hyperreflex spasm, which progressed to respiratory (and cardiac) arrest. No resuscitation was attempted in the clinic. The child was rushed to a nearby hospital but was declared 'brought dead'. The parents filed a complaint, and an FIR was registered under Section 304A. The pedodontist and anaesthetist were arrested but subsequently released on bail.

A criminal case was filed with the following respondents:
1. Pedodontist
2. Anaesthetist
3. Dental clinic

A civil case was filed under the Consumer Protection Act.

A case was filed before the State Dental Council.

The case is still ongoing.

Anecdote 5

An apparently healthy child was treated for a pulpotomy or RCT in a dental clinic. Routine informed consent was obtained. The pedodontist was performing the procedure under routine local anaesthesia. The child, who was responsive at the beginning of the procedure, slowly became drowsy. The dentist did not notice this. Subsequently, the child voided her bladder. The dentist then tried to rouse the child, but she was unresponsive and could not be awakened. The dentist had no monitoring device. He felt a very feeble pulse and immediately stopped the procedure and tried to move the patient to a nearby pediatrician. The child was declared 'brought dead'. Criminal and civil cases were filed. The autopsy was inconclusive for any findings. A complaint was lodged by the parents against the dentist and clinic. An FIR was registered under Section 304A. No arrest was made in view of Supreme Court rulings in the Jacob Mathew Case.

Civil and statutory complaints were made under the Consumer Protection Act and with the State Dental Council, respectively.

Decisions are pending for above three anecdotes.

Anecdote 6

A middle-aged man was seen by a dentist with a toothache and mobility of the upper teeth. He gave no history of any medical problems when asked verbally. The patient was in severe pain, and the dentist gave him antibiotics and analgesics, asking him to report the next day.

The patient returned the next day complaining of persistent pain in the teeth, upper jaw, and eye. The dentist extracted the mobile tooth or teeth under local anesthesia. The patient returned the following day with a significant swelling in the midface, suggestive of cellulitis. The dentist referred him to a physician, where he was admitted. Routine blood tests revealed that he had diabetes mellitus with a blood glucose value of 500 mg/dl. The physician instituted empirical intravenous antibiotics and insulin. A PNS X-ray revealed pan-sinusitis. The patient also had pus discharged through the nose. He was thereafter referred to an ENT surgeon. While under the care of the ENT surgeon, he developed a reduction in visual acuity in one eye. The cellulitis had by then subsided, but his vision was deteriorating. He was then sent to an ophthalmic hospital, where he was diagnosed as having orbital apex syndrome secondary to infection, causing blindness in one eye. The specialists blamed the dentist for having extracted the tooth without ascertaining his diabetic status.

The patient sent a legal notice and filed a case in the District Consumer Court for ₹10 lakhs. The Consumer Court did not uphold the case as negligence. This was managed with some good legal responses. However, an out-of-court settlement with compensation was paid as a humanitarian gesture to cover medical costs!

Anecdote 7

A patient was seen by a dentist for a deep cavity in a molar tooth. The dentist suggested root canal treatment, which was readily accepted by the patient. The patient was very apprehensive and fidgety, moving throughout the procedure. The dentist then lost one of the instruments in the mouth. He examined it and failed to locate it intra-orally. He referred the patient to a general surgeon for an opinion. A diagnostic radiograph was performed, which revealed that the instrument was in the stomach. The general surgeon decided to retrieve it through an endoscopic procedure. However, the patient was very uncooperative during the procedure, and the food in his stomach also made it impossible to complete the retrieval. Despite assurance and observation, the patient sought further treatment at a specialty hospital in a neighbouring city. By the next day, the instrument had travelled further down the gastro-intestinal tract without causing any problem. One week later, the instrument had moved out of the body, and it was concluded that he had passed it.

The patient nevertheless filed a civil case with the consumer protection forum. The dentist had good legal assistance and argued that for medical negligence, there should be an injury. In the absence of a significant injury and because he sought further treatment against the advice of specialists, the forum was not inclined to find a deficiency of service. The case was withdrawn.